American Publishing Health Book Series

New And Natural Ways To

Lower Your Blood Pressure, Cholesterol And Stress

By

Greg Tyler
Christina Tyler

AMERICAN PUBLISHING CORPORATION
© 1997. ALL RIGHTS RESERVED

IMPORTANT NOTICE

This manual is intended as a reference volume only, not as a
medical guide or a reference for self treatment. You should
always seek competent medical advice from a doctor if you
suspect a problem.
This book is intended as educational device to keep you
informed of the latest medical knowledge. It is not intended
to serve as a substitute for changing the treatment advice of
your doctor. You should never make medical changes without first consulting your doctor.

Additional copies of this book may be purchased directly
from the publisher. To order, please enclose $23.95 plus $3
postage and handling. Send to:

*NEW AND NATURAL WAYS TO LOWER YOUR BLOOD
PRESSURE, CHOLESTEROL AND STRESS*

American Publishing Corporation
Book Distribution Center
Post Box 15196
Montclair, CA 91763

Printed in the United States of America

0 9 8 7 6 5 4 3 2 1

TABLE OF CONTENTS

INTRODUCTION

New And Natural Ways To Lower Your Blood Pressure, Cholesterol And Stress

INTRODUCTION

WHO SHOULD READ THIS BOOK?

You--if you love health and the idea of longevity. If you like adventure. If you're an honest coward (like most of us) and are terrified of dying. Or if you're greedy and want to hang onto everything you've got (except fat), or just want more of everything--days and nights, family pleasures, vacations, sunrises and sunsets.

If you're any or all of these things, read the pages that follow. But:

Warning: This book could be hazardous--not to your health, which may already be in jeopardy, but hazardous to your complacency.

Why? Because we've packed a good deal of frightening data between these covers, up-to-the-minute data concerning coronary heart disease, the worst mass killer of our century. A killer that, statistics show, could have you high on its hit list.

If this sounds like we're trying to scare you, you're right. We think a little fright-for-your-life will help you fight for your life--and help provide the motivation you need to defeat this killer.

Because you can win the fight against heart disease.

Remember, we called it the worst mass killer of our century? That's because, oddly enough, this deadly disease was far less prevalent during earlier eras. This is not just an interesting historical sidelight. It has immense implications. Either we're doing something wrong now we didn't used to do as a people, or not doing something right we used to do, or both. (Much more about this later.)

The heartening fact is, there are many things we can all do to combat heart disease and its debilitating effects--atherosclerosis, heart attacks and stroke. And that's the special sermon of this book. Once we've scared you a bit, we want to share with you a wealth of health secrets, secrets not only to stop coronary disease in its insidious tracks and reverse its effects, but put you on the road to an unsurpassed sense of wellness and longevity. (We've also included highlights and critiques of current cholesterol-reducing diets.)

We don't claim any particular originality for these secrets (though we do offer original ways to maximize benefits). Most of these ideas are the hard-won fruits of nutritional science or mainstream medical science.

Which brings us to a very important disclaimer: Everything we recommend in these pages should be considered as a supplemental (or complementary) to a physician's advice and treatment. This is especially true if your cholesterol is in the danger zone (see "Getting a Fix on Cholesterol Risk" in Chapter One.)

Now, before we go any farther, here's a sneak preview of some "secrets" we'll discuss at length later on:

9 Easy Steps to Heart Health

1. Exercise.

2. Become a thin person.

3. Lower carbohydrate and total sugars.

4. Eat bran and drink more good water.

5. Avoid constipation.

6. Eat several small meals daily.

7. Eat a good across-the-board food supplement.

8. Add enzymes to your diet.

9. Use B-3 (niacin) to restore your full blood- stream.

You'll find the amplification on each item (and many, many others) in subsequent chapters. In fact, you'll find bits and pieces of these "cholesterol cures" scattered throughout.

But right now you need to learn more about your wonderful heart, and how to keep it, and you, happy.

Greg & Christina Tyler

I. 20TH-CENTURY PLAGUE

HOW LONG SHOULD YOUR HEART LAST?

If you think 70 years is pretty good for a heart to keep on beating, you're way off. Actually twice 70 years is closer!

Sounds like science fiction perhaps? It's not. Many researchers have come to the conclusion that the heart is built to last much longer than our expected life span. In fact, it is just possible that your heart should last for about 120 to 140 years! (Scientists arrive at this amazing figure along several lines of logic--historic, zoologic and experimental.)

Alas, this perpetual motion machine rarely gets a chance to operate the way it was meant to. Later on we'll discuss ways to restore the heart to full functionality--its "factory warranty." But right now it's important to focus on why the average American heart endures only about half its possible lifespan--70 years. And why many hearts give out after only around 60 years, some 50 or even less, and why many start degenerating much sooner than that.

The short and unavoidable answer as to why the average heart doesn't last longer is that we do things to it which hamper its optimum function and survival.

We'll going to talk about those heart-rending things we all do to ourselves and tell you how to stop doing them.

But first, we need to focus on the frightening dimensions of heart disease and heart attacks--the hows and whys and how manys.

THE KILLER WITHIN

There is absolute agreement today--from experts and laymen alike--that heart disease, in all its virulent varieties, is our nation's number one killer. There can be no disputing that this disease is on a rampage through our adult population, and that everyone who values his or her life--and especially those with "high-risk" profiles--needs to take the most immediate and effective steps possible to prevent it from striking, to treat it when it strikes, and, if possible, to reverse its deadly effects.

Unfortunately, there is widespread disagreement about what constitutes the most effective preventatives and countermeasures to heart attacks and heart disease. The medical establishment continues to pretend that it has the only revealed truth, but even those haughty bastions are beginning to crumble.

Such publications of medical correctness as the Harvard Heart Letter and the Journal of the American Medical Association are having to acknowledge (belatedly and begrudgingly) the amazing breakthroughs in cholesterol and blood-pressure reduction through non-medical modes--especially nutrition (vitamins, minerals, herbs, etc.). These mainstream journals try to minimize these documented and often miraculous results, but they can no longer pretend that there is no alternative to physician-dispensed prescription medications and the typical low-cholesterol diet regimen.

In fact, the number of alternative remedies and treatments is growing daily, with wide divergence among the various proponents. Just in the area of heart-healthful diets, there are those who recommend high-carbohydrates and others who maintain that high carbs actually increase dangerous cholesterol levels. While the majority of nutritionists may adhere to the gospel of low-fat foods, there is no shortage of reformers who do not--and who have dramatic evidence to back up their positions.

In this book we will survey all these various opinions on heart disease treatment--both establishment and alternative--with a view to helping you, the reader, reach the best-informed opinion. It is, after all, a matter of life and death--your life or your death--and nothing less than an in-depth examination of the matter will do.

We do not pretend to be neutral. While we take a back seat to no one in our appreciation of the miracles of modern medicine, we are keenly aware of its shortcomings--particularly its failure (or refusal) to recognize and incorporate non-medical advances.

By "modern medicine" we mean the medical establishment. But thousands upon thousands of individual physicians have deserted the anti-nutritional orthodoxy, and more and more are doing so every day. Indeed, many of the breakthrough works on alternative procedures for reducing cholesterol and hypertension have been accomplished by medical professionals.

We think you will agree that the results they are getting in combatting heart attacks and heart disease are both exciting and encouraging for all of us. In fact, though coronary statistics continue to be grim, never before has there been so much cause for optimism--optimism that we can win this battle against our number one killer.

Before we get too optimistic, however, let's have a look at those grim statistics. It's important to know thy enemy, after all.

WHO'S AT RISK FROM HEART ATTACKS?

The short and scary answer is that everyone is potentially at risk. Despite all the publicity for other calamitous diseases--all forms of cancer, AIDS, and so on--heart disease remains Public Enemy No. 1--by a wide margin, America's greatest killer.

Every year just in the U.S. a half a million people die suddenly, while a million more die from diseases of the heart and blood vessels. That's almost two deaths per minute, about equal to the number of people killed from all other causes combined!

However, some people are at even greater risk than others. There are certain factors known to increase a person's susceptibility to heart attacks and heart disease.

GOOD NEWS/BAD NEWS ABOUT HEART DISEASE

The surprising good news about heart disease is that the rate actually is declining--the probability of dying from cardiovascular disease declined by 24.5%

from 1982 to 1992, and the risk today is less than half what it was in 1950.

The bad news: cardiovascular disease remains the number one cause of death in the U.S., as it has been every year since 1900 (except one, 1918, when a devastating influenza epidemic occurred). Today, cardiovascular disease accounts for about 42% of all deaths in the U.S. Nearly a quarter of the U.S. population has some form of cardiovascular disease, and more than 11 million have coronary artery disease (according to the American Heart Association).

CORONARY RISK FACTORS

There have been many studies of this--the most famous being a long-term investigation of residents in the Massachusetts community of Framingham. All of these studies have agreed in isolating several factors that definitely increase a person's chances of developing coronary disease.

Unfortunately, three of these risk factors can't be changed:

1.   Age--over 45 for men, over 55 for women.

2.   Gender--men are at greater risk than women.

3. Genetics--having a family history of heart attack or sudden death (father or brother stricken before age 55 or a mother or sister before 65).

But--the good news--eight risk factors can be changed, or at least controlled. They are:

1. Smoking

2. Lack of exercise

3. High blood cholesterol (high total cholesterol and high LDL cholesterol, about which a great deal more later)

4. Low HDL cholesterol (also to be discussed later)

5. High blood pressure (or hypertension)

6. Diabetes

7. Being overweight

8. Loneliness, depression, stress (and other psychological factors)

SHORT PEOPLE--AT GREATER RISK OF HEART DISEASE?

A couple years back there was epidemiological data suggesting that shorter people have a higher heart disease risk. The news got a lot of publicity--and certainly scared many people of shorter stature.

The initial study was of 5,296 men and 7,735 women who participated in a national project called the First National Health and Nutrition Examination Survey from 1971 to 1975.

Average height of the women in this study was 5'3", while the men averaged 5'8". Among both men and women, shorter people tended to have more risk factors for coronary artery disease. Cholesterol levels were not correlated with height, but tall people were less likely to be obese and to have high blood pressure or diabetes.

During an average follow-up of 13 years, the researchers found an elevated rate of heart disease in shorter people. However, after adjusting for other risk factors for heart disease, such as age and education, height alone was not associated with risk of heart attack or death.

These data suggest that shorter people are at no increased risk of a heart attack or heart disease, but do highlight the fact that short people have a high rate of problems such as obesity and hypertension. Fortunately, these factors can be controlled through changes in lifestyle and the use of antihypertensive medications.

VISIBLE INDICATOR OF HEART ATTACK RISK?

Over the years many doctors have noticed that a diagonal crease in the earlobe of patients was much more pronounced among their heart attack patients. Several subsequent studies, including one at the Mayo Clinic, have confirmed this unlikely indicator of coronary artery disease. While there are too many variables for the Crease Factor to be established as scientifically sound, it is at least one more diagnostic tool for the cardiovascular specialist. There has been no shortage of theories attempting to explain it, but until there is more evidence, the idea remains only a very intriguing speculation.

EMOTIONAL RISK FACTORS, TRUE OR FALSE?

Many people feel intuitively that certain negative emotions can help bring on a heart attack, emotions like rage and high-anxiety. The image of the agitated person collapsing during a heart attack is familiar from movies, but how often does this happen in real life? Well, medical science has finally gotten around to asking this question and seeing if there's any truth to these popular beliefs. The results are surprising:

* Anger and Heart Attacks

Researchers at New England Deaconess Hospital and Harvard Medical School conducted a series of investigations of what factors actually trigger heart attacks. A research team interviewed 1,623 patients who had just had coronaries, asking about the frequency of anger during the previous year and during the hours before their attack.

The survey found that 8% of the patients reported episodes of anger the day prior to their heart attack, and 2.4% had experienced angry episodes in the two hours prior to their heart attack. Analysis indicated that episodes of anger more than doubled the risk of a heart attack for about two hours; after that, the period of danger passed.

Since only 2.4% of the patients who had heart attacks reported anger in the two hours prior to their events, the study suggests that anger is not a major public health problem or a main trigger of heart attacks. But the findings do confirm theories that anger and other psychological stress might affect blood clotting or other factors that can lead to heart attacks in susceptible individuals.

* Anxiety and Heart Disease

Data linking anxiety and heart attack risk were reported in a study of 2,280 Boston men over a 32-year period. Compared with the men who reported no symptoms of anxiety, those who reported two or more symptoms showed three times the risk of dying from heart disease and a nearly sixfold increase in risk of sudden death.

Note: The increased risk associated with anxiety was at least partially due to the fact that the men with more anxiety were more likely to smoke cigarettes. But even after adjusting for smoking and other coronary risk factors, the results strongly indicated a higher rate of heart problems for anxious people.

(To learn about combatting anxiety, see Chapter Six, "Escape From Stress.")

Both studies--of anger and anxiety--point to a link between a patient's psychological state and heart disease.

ASPIRIN TO THE RESCUE

Many clinical studies have found that aspirin can decrease the dangerous effect of anger. There seems to be only a slight trend toward increased risk after anger episodes for patients who reported regular use of aspirin. However, among non-users of aspirin, anger episodes appear to nearly triple the risk of heart attack for two hours.

In 1995 the British Medical Journal published a study in which more than 140,000 patients had taken aspirin or other anti-clotting drugs in an attempt to prevent heart attack, stroke or death. The voluminous findings were boiled down to a single strong recommendation:

Almost anyone who has ever had a heart attack or stroke, or who suffers from angina, or has undergone coronary artery bypass surgery, should take one-half to one aspirin tablet daily--unless allergic to the drug.

Caution: Because of possible bleeding complications, those at low risk for heart disease or stroke should probably forgo the daily aspirin, or take reduced-strength "baby aspirin."

The researchers speculated that if their advice were adopted by high-risk patients worldwide, 100,000 deaths and perhaps 200,000 non-fatal strokes and heart attacks could be prevented annually.

MYTHS AND MISCONCEPTIONS ABOUT HEART DISEASE

Many of us think we know certain things about heart disease that simply aren't true. Here's a list of common fallacies:

1. Heart disease is a bigger problem for men than women.

Men are at greater risk, as mentioned above. But in terms of sheer numbers, more women than men die annually of the disease. Cancer is fatal to more males than females, however.

2. Heart disease is mainly dangerous for older people.

Deaths are more common among older people, but about 5% of all heart attacks occur in people under age 65. Of all the people who die from cardiovascular disease, almost 40% are under age 75. Thus, more than a third of the deaths due to diseases of the heart and blood vessels can be considered premature.

3. Heart-disease primarily affects white males.

Cardiovascular disease is the leading cause of deaths for blacks at all ages. The death rate, in fact, is nearly 50% higher than the rate for white males. And the rate of cardiovascular death for black females is 69% higher than for white females.

4. It's OK to wait for symptoms of heart problems before acting to control risk factors.

This frightening fallacy will be discussed in detail below under "silent heart attacks." The scary fact is that for 48% of men and 63% of women who die suddenly of coronary artery disease, there was no previous evidence of heart problems. Despite medical advances, sudden death is the first sign of heart disease in about one-half of all heart attacks.

5. The stressful life of the executive causes heart attacks.

Perhaps, but hypertension and heart attacks are more common among people with lower educational and income levels.

6. Because of anti-tobacco education, smoking will soon cease to be a health problem.

Smoking has declined the U.S. since 1965 by more than a third, but about 28% of U.S. men and 25% of U.S. women still smoke, and nearly one-fifth of deaths from cardiovascular illnesses are attributable to smoking. Doctors now estimate that smoking doubles the risk of having a heart attack.

7. For the elderly the biggest health problems are cancer and dementia like Alzheimer's.

Cancer and dementia are indeed cause for concern as we grow older, but heart failure is the single most frequent cause of hospitalization for people over age 65.

THE TICKING TIME BOMB

Silent heart attacks, also known as sudden cardiac death (SCD), can strike anyone without warning--as mentioned previously, 500,000 a year.

They strike without warning because the victim in many cases has had no pre-existing symptoms, or is unaware of any symptoms.

And that is really worth stressing:

* Some people who have heart attacks have not previously sought medical attention because they simply did not recognize their symptoms as worrisome.

* Others may not have had any symptoms at all.

* Others actually experience heart attacks and don't recognize them as such, and therefore do not get medical help.

These unrecognized heart attacks can lead to sudden cardiac arrest--which too often means sudden death. Even if these unrecognized attacks do not cause any immediate consequences, they do have longer-term importance. Reason? People who have had one heart attack are at high risk for having another.

HOW COMMON ARE 'SILENT' HEART ATTACKS?

A recent study from Iceland provided insight into unrecognized, or "silent" coronaries.

Out of more than 9,000 men surveyed since 1967, 237 were found to have had heart attacks--and more than a third had experienced unrecognized heart attacks. Though almost no one under 40 had a silent heart attack, more than 5% of the patients aged 75-79 had had an unrecognized heart attack. (See MORE ON SILENT HEART ATTACKS below.)

The chances of living 10 years after an unrecognized heart attack was 49%, compared with 62% for those with an recognized heart attack. So silent heart attacks are not less serious than recognized heart attacks. In fact, those who have had a silent attack seem to fare worse, perhaps because they are less likely to receive treatments shown to improve survival after a heart attack.

Conclusion: Those middle-aged and older should be evaluated by their physician immediately if they even suspect they have symptoms of a heart attack. And those with risk factors for a heart attack should undergo an electrocardiogram every few years so the doctor can specifically check for evidence of a heart attack.

HOW HEART ATTACKS HAPPEN

To understand the dangerous and degenerative process leading to heart attacks, we need to first discuss one of the main culprits--cholesterol. Or at least the culprit known as "bad" cholesterol (yes, there is also "good" cholesterol).

Cholesterol, which is produced in the liver, is a fatty substance in the outer lining of body cells. It is carried in the bloodstream to the cells by special proteins called "lipoproteins." Cholesterol, which has the properties of an oil, can't dissolve in blood without lipoproteins.

The two major lipoproteins are low-density lipoprotein (LDL) and high-density lipoprotein (HDL). LDL lipoprotein, the prime carrier of blood cholesterol, is often called "bad" cholesterol, because elevated LDL cholesterol is associated with an increased risk of coronary heart disease.

HDL lipoproteins are mostly protein plus a small amount of cholesterol. HDL lipoproteins remove cholesterol from artery walls, thus protecting us from atherosclerosis. HDL cholesterol, therefore, may be called "good" cholesterol. High HDL cholesterol levels are desirable, while low HDL cholesterol increases the risk of coronary heart disease.

'GOOD' AND 'BAD' CHOLESTEROL

Don't be misled by the "good/bad" labels. The differences have nothing to do with anything "moral," or with virtue or vice, and are as easy to grasp as "softball" and "hardball."

LDL is "bad" only because it's low-density. That means it is "soft fat." The reason this is bad is that blobs of it don't hold together too well in the bloodstream. Have you ever dropped soft butter off your breadknife? That's low density. These globules of fat in the bloodstream stick to arterial walls (not to venous walls). They don't bounce off, they flatten and just smear. They're like a butter-throwing contest. Anybody standing close gets greased.

HDL Cholesterol is fat also, but it's high-density or "hard" fat. These globules of more firm lipoproteins are smaller than the soft ones. When they get jostled against arterial walls, they don't smear, they bound away. That's why they're "good"--because they don't stick.

Merely sticking to the sides of arteries isn't so bad. But when the low-density fats begin to absorb calcium and debris from the bloodstream which is flowing by, they begin a buildup. They harden and become cholesterol deposits, called plaque.

As this build-up occurs, there is, naturally, less room in the artery. Narrow arteries cannot contain as much blood as clean, open ones, and so inside the narrowed lumen (the "open" area inside the blood vessel) the pressure goes up. And increased pressure, just like water in a garden hose, can make the vessel weak and finally burst.

The gradual thickening of the artery walls and narrowing of the arteries lead to a condition known as atherosclerosis. When coronary arteries--the ones supplying blood and oxygen to the heart muscle--are narrowed by atherosclerosis, they can't supply enough blood and oxygen to the heart during exertion.

Atherosclerosis can also lead to formation of a blood clot in the artery, which can cause complete arterial blockage, leading to death of heart muscle (heart attack).

Just as detrimental, the clogged arteries reduce blood flow throughout the body. Thus cells far from the occlusion begin to suffer slow starvation.

This causes discomfort in some people, but not always in everyone. Consequently, the buildup of bad cholesterol inside the arteries can restrict bloodflow, dangerously increase blood pressure and despoil health, and the person hardly realizes he or she is in jeopardy. Quite often, as we've already discussed, nobody learns how great the damage is until the autopsy.

ANOTHER 'BAD' CHOLESTEROL

A recent study has uncovered a little-known form of "bad" cholesterol. Doctors cannot yet measure it reliably, but fear that it may cause early heart disease just as often as its better-known cousins.

This new "baddie," called lipoprotein(a), according to research, may lurk in dangerously high levels in the blood of people whose other cholesterol levels appear normal.

Excess levels of lipoprotein(a), which are particles of protein and fat in the blood, accounted for 10% of all cases of premature heart disease, those occurring before age 55, among the 2,191 men studied, according to the research at the National Heart, Lung and Blood Institute.

The findings were published in the August, 1996, Journal of the American Medical Assn.

The value of knowing an excess Lp(a) level is that it may warn the patient of the need for more aggressive treatment of other traits that also predict heart disease such as smoking, poor diet, high blood pressure and high blood sugar.

ANOTHER 'GOOD' CHOLESTEROL

Usually, genetic mutations mean bad news. But a chance genetic mutation endowed Giovanni Pomaroli, a man from the remote town of Limone, Italy, in 1780, with an unusual protein that prevented cholesterol from building up in his arteries. It allowed him and his descendants to eat massive quantities of fatty foods, smoke to excess, avoid exercise and still live well into their 90s.

More than two-hundred years later, a research team at Cedars-Sinai Medical Center in Los Angeles began using that protein to prevent cholesterol buildup in the arteries of rabbits and mice. that were not naturally endowed with it--and may soon being trying to do the same in humans.

The first likely trial patients will be those who have vascular disease but are not candidates for surgery or angioplasty. Another group would be those who have trouble lowering their cholesterol levels through diet and medication. Patients who have undergone angioplasty to clear their arteries might receive it to prevent further clogging.

The mutant protein, Apo A-1 Milano, was eventually isolated and produced in relatively large quantities by researchers at Pharmacia AB, the Swedish drug company that now supplies it to researchers. Apo A-1 Milano is, in a sense, a biological garbage truck that removes cholesterol from the arteries and dumps it in the body's waste stream.

As we've seen, humans have three types of cholesterol in their blood--the so-called "good cholesterol" (high density lipoprotein, or HDL), "bad cholesterol" (low-density lipoprotein, or LDL) and triglycerides.

LDL carries cholesterol through the body, but it tends to fall apart, leaving plaque deposits on the walls of blood vessels. Triglycerides are converted into LDL. HDL, in contrast, binds cholesterol tightly and carries it to the liver for disposal.

Apo A-1 is a key building block of HDL, and the Milano variant seems to make it work better.

In one study, rats were fed a high-fat diet and scratched the insides of some arteries, a technique that accelerates the formation of atherosclerotic plaque. After plaque built up, the researchers performed angioplasty, in which a balloon is inserted and inflated to compress the plaque. Half the animals received an injection of the Apo A-1 Milano protein before and after angioplasty.

When the team examined both groups three weeks later, they found that rabbits that received the mutant protein had 70% less thickening of the artery wall from plaque buildup. Similar results were found in mice. The gene protects rabbits and mice by both preventing the formation of fatty plaque and also reversing plaque once it's formed.

Meanwhile, researchers are trying to understand precisely how the mutant protein functions in the hope of designing a drug that can do the same thing.

Another possibility is gene therapy. Instead of injecting the Apo A-1 Milano protein into people, researchers would insert the gene for it into the liver, allowing the body to make its own protein. This would basically fool cells into thinking they carry the gene; that will trigger the liver to begin producing the mutant protein.

GETTING A FIX ON CHOLESTEROL RISK

Perhaps you're one of those prudent folks who keeps regular tabs on his or her cholesterol and knows exactly where you fit on the risk-scale. But in case you're not, here are the guidelines suggested by the National Cholesterol Education Program:

TOTAL CHOLESTEROL

Desirable	Less than 200
Borderline High	200 to 239
High	240 or above

LDL CHOLESTEROL

Desirable	Less than 130
Borderline High	130 to 159
High	160 or above

HDL CHOLESTEROL

Desirable	Above 35

(All reading in ml/dl., milligrams/deciliter.)

HEART ATTACKS DEFY LOGIC

Cardiologists have always assumed that a person's chance of having a heart attack rises if there are severe atherosclerotic blockages in a coronary artery--the larger the blockage, the greater the heart-attack risk.

These larger blockages often cause symptoms of chest pain (angina) because the heart is not getting enough blood when the patient exerts himself or herself. Therefore, common sense would dictate that those who develop heart attacks would have several months at least of warning from anginal symptoms.

But recent scientific studies (using angiography, or x-ray of the heart and blood vessels following a dye injection) examining the size of offending blockages have demonstrated that, in fact, the most dangerous blockages are often not the largest. In fact, the average buildup that causes a heart attack blocks only about half the coronary artery's diameter. The more severely blocked arteries--those with 70% or greater--were often not the cause of the heart attack.

These results seem to defy logic. How can smaller blockages be riskier than larger ones? If severe narrowing of an artery is not the cause of a heart attack, what is?

The answer lies in the nature of the plaques that make up the blockages.

TURNING THE MICROSCOPE ON PLAQUES

Plaques are made of cholesterol, fats, fibrous tissue, and white blood cells, all deposited in the artery walls over time. But these deposits can vary in consistency, some being prone to rupture while others are quite stable. The "mix" of these kinds of plaques appears to play a critical role in determining who is likely to have a heart attacks.

* Stable Plaques vs. Unstable Ones

Stable plaques grow gradually over the years, which gives time for blood flow to develop in new arteries, called collateral vessels. These collateral vessels bypass the clogged artery and bring the life-giving blood and oxygen to the heart. Even if these stable plaques become quite large, they are rarely responsible for a heart attack. In fact, arteries may become completely blocked by stable plaques, while the heart remains healthy because of collateral vessels.

Time, the ally of those with stable plaques,

becomes the enemy when plaques are unstable. Cardiologists now suspect that nearly all heart attacks are caused by the rupture of these unstable plaques, made up primarily of fats and white blood cells. The thin fibrous cap on these plaques can be weakened by the white cells, which attack and digest parts of it. High blood pressure, high cholesterol levels and smoking also make these plaques more vulnerable to rupture.

These plaques can rupture suddenly and without warning. The rupture then triggers a cascade of events: the plaque material spills into the artery. This can cause blood clots, which in turn block the blood supply to the heart, destroying a large part of the heart muscle.

This is a heart attack.

MORE ON SILENT HEART ATTACKS

This helps to explain why a sudden heart attack can strike without warning, or without previous symptoms. Typically, victims of silent heart attacks have considered themselves perfectly healthy--they may have exercised faithfully for years, and never have experienced chest pain.

That's because, until the moment of rupture, the diseased coronary artery has delivered sufficient blood to the heart. That "good news" turns disastrous when the plaque ruptures and the coronary artery become clogged, because no collateral vessels have developed to bypass the artery and deliver the usual blood supply.

WHICH ATTACKS ARE MOST LIKELY FATAL?

There have been dramatic improvement in treating heart-attack victims--once the patient reaches the hospital. For instance, balloon angioplasties can widen arteries and thrombolysis can dissolve clots. Using these methods, physicians save more than 90% of those who get to the hospital alive. But around half of those who have heart attacks every year--approximately 250,000 people in the U.S.--die before they arrive at the hospital. Most of those are victims of so-called "silent" attacks.

Are there any warning signs these people might have detected?

Yes, according to Americans Heart Association. They advise people to call 911 or the local emergency medical service number immediately if they ever experience any of the following symptoms:

* Pain spreading to the shoulders, neck or arms.

* Uncomfortable pressure, fullness, squeezing, or pain in the center of the chest lasting more than a few minutes.

* Chest discomfort with lightheadedness, fainting, sweating, nausea or shortness of breath.

SPOTTING 'UNSTABLE' CLOTS

"Hot spots" in clogged arteries may warn of an imminent heart attack, U.S. doctors reported in May, 1996. They said their findings could lead to the development of screening techniques that could warn patients most in danger.

Many heart attacks are caused by a condition known as atherosclerosis, when fatty deposits in the arteries break off and form a clot that blocks blood flow. Some of the deposits, or plaques, have a thin covering of cells, but others are more unstable and have inflammatory cells inside.

Dr. Ward Casscells and colleagues at the University of Texas medical school in Houston decided to see if there was a way to detect the more unstable deposits.

They examined the arteries of 48 patients, and found the unstable ones showed a higher temperature. In fact, 37 percent of the plaques were significantly warmer and were associated with the inflammatory cells.

In a report in the Lancet medical journal, they said their findings could be used to find a test for the "hot spots" so doctors could quickly treat patients most at risk.

CAN 'UNSTABLE' PLAQUES BE STABILIZED?

Not only is this a good question, it's precisely the task that many cardiologists are working feverishly to accomplish. They are trying to understand why plaques become unstable in the first place, so they'll have a better grasp of whether they can be transformed into stable ones.

One suggested technique has been to destroy the unstable or vulnerable lesions with balloon angioplasty or other catheter devices before they get to the point of rupturing. But to do this, cardiologists must first be able to recognize them, and current angiographic technology does not yet distinguish unstable from stable lesions.

So, for the time being, the most realistic approach seems to lie in cholesterol reduction or control. Studies in animals indicate that when blood levels of cholesterol are lowered, fat content of plaques also falls--increasing the stability of the plaques.

One benefit of lowering blood cholesterol may be removal of lipid from all of the plaques in the arteries, particularly the most unstable ones.

The question remains, however, how best to reduce the "bad" LDL cholesterol. Unfortunately, the traditional medical remedies, such as cholesterol-lowering medication plus a diet low in animal fats, have not led to any dramatic reductions in these grim statistics.

NEW BIRTH-CONTROL PILLS MAY INCREASE RISK OF BLOOD CLOTS

Back in the '60s, women who used oral contraceptives, also known as birth-control pills, were plagued by complications, including blood clots. Fortunately, cardiovascular problems from these medications were reduced when manufacturers decreased the estrogen content.

In recent years, "third-generation" birth-control pills have emerged that include newer progestins, which are intended to further reduce the risk of cardiovascular complications. Unfortunately, a recent series of studies link these third-generation pills to an increased risk of blood clots in the veins of the women who take them. Three large studies all detected approximately a doubling of risk of blood-clot complications in women using third-generation compared with other oral contraceptives.

An accompanying study indicates that the risk may be especially large in women who have never been pregnant or who are carriers of a genetic marker (called a factor V Leiden mutation). Nevertheless, among medical authorities the question remains whether women should switch from newer agents back to the older contraceptives.

However, the increase in risk of dying is estimated to be only one per year for every million women using third-generation instead of older drugs. Furthermore, the presence of a progestin in these pills may offer other long-term benefits to women that offset the increase in blood-dot risk. So the jury remains out on whether these new agents are an advance--or a step backward.

TRIGLYCERIDES AND CORONARY HEART DISEASE

Triglycerides are the major form of fat, the form in which fat is stored in the body. They come from food as well as being produced in the body.

High triglyceride levels (greater than 200) are also linked to a higher occurrence of coronary heart disease. Triglyceride levels are influenced by recent fat and alcohol intake, and therefore should be measured after fasting for at least 12 hours. In fact, a period of abstinence from alcohol is advised before testing for triglycerides.

Like cholesterol, triglycerides are measured in milligrams/deciliter. Here are the National Cholesterol Education Program's guidelines for triglyceride levels:

200   Borderline high

400   High

1,000   Very high

Markedly high triglyceride levels (greater than 500mg/dl) can cause pancreatitis--inflammation of the pancreas. Therefore, these high levels should be treated aggressively with low fat diets and medications, if needed.

TRIGLYCERIDES AND WOMEN

High triglycerides may play a more important role in women than in men, according to some cardiologists. Triglycerides are also higher in people with uncontrolled diabetes, itself a risk factor for heart disease.

Triglycerides are essential to life. But consuming too many triglycerides can cause the body to make too much cholesterol. Some studies have concluded that there is no direct association between triglyceride levels and cardiovascular risk. But other research has shown a significant association between the two.

In the Framingham Heart Study, high triglycerides in association with low HDL cholesterol were found to be an independent predictor of coronary heart disease in men and women over age 50.

Researchers in Norway analyzed triglyceride levels in 24,535 middle-age women and found that as triglyceride readings increased, so did deaths related to coronary heart disease-as well as deaths from all causes. The researchers found no relationship between triglycerides and mortality in 25,058 men, however.

Researchers at Johns Hopkins University School of Medicine in Baltimore examined the relationship between cardiovascular disease and various blood fat measurements (total, HDL and LDL cholesterol and triglycerides) in about 1,400 women ages 50 to 69. Over a 14-year period, high triglycerides were associated with an increased risk of dying of heart disease.

These researchers concluded that elevated triglycerides are an independent predictor of death from cardiovascular disease in women.

HOW HIGH-BLOOD PRESSURE INCREASES HEART ATTACK RISK

Those with uncontrolled high blood pressure are three times as likely to develop coronary artery disease, statistics show, six times as likely to develop congestive heart failure, and seven times as likely to have a stroke. Hypertension is considered the single most important risk factor for congestive heart failure, contributing to 91% of the cases of the disease that have developed over the last two decades.

Despite widespread awareness of the risk of hypertension, average blood pressures have been increasing rather than declining, according to Dr. William B. Kannel of the Boston University School of Medicine. He has found that the average blood pressure among adults age 30 to 65 has increased by about 20/10 millimeters of mercury over the last four decades.

New And Natural Ways To Lower Your Blood Pressure, Cholesterol And Stress

Over half of the Americans who have high blood pressure are unaware that they have it. Another 17 percent, who know they have it, are not on therapy. And 27 percent are treated but not adequately or are not dependable in taking their medications. Only one in five Americans with high blood pressure have their disease under control. This means millions are at risk for stroke and heart attack.

How much is "high"?

People are considered to have hypertension if their systolic blood pressure is at least 140 mm Hg or their diastolic blood pressure is at least 90 mm Hg, or if they take antihypertensive medication. By these measuring sticks, about 50 million Americans have high blood pressure.

Systolic blood pressure is the higher of two numbers in a blood-pressure reading. It shows the pressure in the arteries when the heart contracts.

Diastolic pressure is the lower of the two numbers. It measures pressure when the heart is relaxed.

Certain factors raise the chance of having high blood pressure. We've already noted that clogged arteries cause elevated blood pressure. But there are other causative factors:

* Carrying too much weight is a critical one: high blood pressure is at least twice as great in overweight populations as in those non-overweight.

* Lack of exercise also increases blood pressure, which usually falls after the patient begins a regular exercise program. (Ironically, vigorous physical activity actually raises blood pressure, but this kind is brief--and, in fact, probably strengthens arteries and heart against these very infirmities.

* Age and race can influence whether or not a person is prone to high blood pressure: the older people get, the higher pressure tends to be, and black people are more likely to have high blood pressure than white people.

* Taking in too much salt or alcohol increases the chance of having high blood pressure and can cause many other adverse health effects. (There is, however, some scientific controversy on this issue. See below.)

* Stress can also causes high blood pressure.

CLASSIFICATION OF BLOOD PRESSURE

Category	Systolic (mm Hg)	Diastolic (mm Hg)
Optimal	under 120	under 80
Normal	under 130	under 85
High normal	130-139	85-89
Hypertension		
Stage 1 (Mild)	140-159	90-99
Stage 2 (Moderate)	160-179	100-109
Stage 3 (Severe)	180-209	110-119
Stage 4 (Very Severe)	210 or more	120 or more

SOME DRUGLESS BLOOD-PRESSURE 'DOWNERS'

The common strategies for lowering hypertension are, as you might expect, attempts to undo or reverse the causative factors listed above:

* Regular physical activity

* Weight loss

* Cutting down salt intake

* Decreased alcohol consumption

Let's take those one by one:

* Regular physical activity: For most people with high blood pressure, 30-45 minutes of brisk walking three to five times per week will be beneficial. Regular aerobic physical activity (which will usually help with weight loss) can reduce systolic blood pressure in hypertensive patients by approximately 10 mm Hg.

Some good aerobic activities: walking, running, cycling, swimming, stair-climbing. Make a point of exercising before any stressful event. This will help bring down your blood pressure during the event.

Caution: weight-lifting can increase blood pressure.

* Weight loss: In clinical studies, patients with hypertension who lost an average of 23 pounds decreased their systolic and diastolic blood pressure by 11 and 8 mm Hg, respectively. In fact, a reduction in blood pressure can occur with a weight loss as small as 10 pounds.

* Cutting down salt intake: A high salt intake does not always cause hypertension. (See following section on genetics.) Similarly, a reduction does not always control hypertension. Still, a reduction in sodium intake to about 2,000 to 2,400 mg. per day (instead of the average intake of around 4,000 to 5,000 mg.) generally lowers both systolic and diastolic blood pressure by about 5 mm Hg. (One teaspoon of table salt has 2,300 milligrams of sodium.) Patients with hypertension should try to stay away from processed foods in general and should read all package labels carefully.

* Decreased alcohol consumption: People who drink three or more alcoholic beverages a day are almost twice as likely as teetotalers to develop hypertension. By cutting back to one drink per day, hypertensive individuals who were heavy drinkers can bring their pressure down.

Bonus: Cigarettes may not hype your blood pressure, but they work in combination with elevated pressure to increase risk of cardiovascular disease. So if you smoke, there's one more reason to stop.

HOW ANTIOXIDANTS LOWER BLOOD PRESSURE

The blood vessels are lined with a layer of endothelial cells that secrete relaxing factors, which cause the vessels to expand, thus lowering blood pressure. One such relaxing factor is nitric oxide. Nitric oxide is rapidly inactivated by a free radical called the superoxide radicals. Increasing your antioxidant protection reduces the number of superoxide radicals, which spares nitric oxide and allows the blood vessels to expand. The net result is lower blood pressure.

GENETICS: PRIME CAUSE OF HIGH-BLOOD PRESSURE?

Scientists are beginning to focus on the genetics of high blood pressure, or hypertension, a condition which affects up to one in five people in the industrialized world.

Research has recently isolated 10 genetic mutations linked to hypertension, all of them involving how kidneys absorb salt and water. In fact, there is an emerging scientific consensus that most cases of hypertension are caused by a combination of genetic and environmental factors, including diet and salt intake. As mentioned above, not everyone who eats salt develops high blood pressure. The reason apparently, is genetic.

The goal of this research is to identify the genetic susceptibility to high blood pressure. Then, patients at risk can be identified and helped before they develop the disease.

When physicians learn more about genetic susceptibility, they'll know which people need to cut back on salt intake, and which do not.

MORE ON THE SALT CONTROVERSY

A University of Toronto study reported in the Journal of the American Medical Association (May 22, 1996) showed that reducing salt in the diet did not lower blood pressure in people who were already healthy, and had only minor effects in those with high blood pressure.

The study , by Dr. Alexander Logan, also argued that avoiding salt can in some cases be harmful, particularly among people who exercise a great deal.

"We can no longer accept on blind faith that restricting salt intake is harmless," Dr. Logan said.

The National Institutes of Health recommends that Americans consume no more than six grams of salt per day, the equivalent of about one teaspoon. The American Heart Assn. recommends a limit of three grams per day. The average American, however, consumes 15 to 20 grams of salt per day, much of it in processed foods.

CUTTING HYPERTENSION WITH SALT SUBSTITUTES

Researchers from the Netherlands decided to test a nutritional theory that adding potassium and magnesium to the diet can lower blood pressure. They took 100 men and women between the ages of 55 and 75 with untreated hypertension. At table and for cooking, half used a special mineral salt containing 40% common salt with the remainder potassium chloride and magnesium salts. The other 50 participants used common salt (sodium chloride).

Those who used mineral salt did not report any lack of saltiness in their food. The only significant difference was noted by the medical evaluators at the conclusion of the test. Those who had used the mineral salt had an average decline in systolic and diastolic blood pressure of 8 and 3 mm Hg respectively, compared with those who used common salt.

Conclusion: If you have hypertension, consider switching from common salt to a low-sodium, high-potassium, high-magnesium salt.

RISKS/BENEFITS OF BLOOD-PRESSURE AND CHOLESTEROL DRUGS

Most people take it for granted that, along with diet and exercise, the best way to control high blood pressure and high cholesterol is to take hypertensive medication. And, unfortunately, too many doctors reach too easily for their prescription pad and the drug cabinet.

But informed opinion on this is shifting. More and more doctors and health professionals are coming to the realization that, except in very dangerous conditions, medication should be the remedy of last resort, not the first. There are too many dramatic results of bringing down bad cholesterol and hypertension through what doctors call "non-pharmacological interventions"--and thereby avoiding dangerous side effects.

But before we discuss these natural solutions, we need to examine more closely the dangers associated with the drugs currently being prescribed for hypertension and cholesterol.

Notes:

_____

_____

_____

_____

_____

_____

_____

II. WHAT YOU MUST KNOW ABOUT CARDIOVASCULAR DRUGS

ARE ALL 'DRUGS' BAD FOR YOU?

Absolutely not. The right drug can save your life. The examples would fill many books--and testimonials abound. So let us be clear: Neither this chapter, nor any other part of this book, should be construed as a condemnation of manmade drugs or of the pharmaceutical industry.

The assertion we are making is an obvious one, one with which most physicians would agree. Drugs focus on treating symptoms, not underlying causes, of an illness. They attempt to affect physical functions, not onl helping the body adjust its own functioning. And, as we all know, pharmaceuticals almost invariably cause side effects. At best, these effects can be unpleasant. At worst, they can be terribly injurious--sometimes worse than the original malady.

SO YOU'RE ALREADY TAKING A CARDIO-VASCULAR MEDICATION

Physicians regularly prescribe cholesterol-lowering medications for those with high LDL cholesterol (greater than 190). These medications are also widely dispensed to those with LDL cholesterol greater than 160 and two or more coronary heart disease risk factors.

For patients with either angina or a prior heart attack, total blood and LDL cholesterol is often treated with medication at lower levels. For example, drug therapy is usually recommended for LDL above 130.

If your doctor feels you fall into one of these high-risk categories and has prescribed medication, by all means keep taking it. You may find your current prescription listed below, with various nasty or scary side effects, and may want to simply quit. Don't do it!

By all means, do study this book, investigate alternative therapies and remedies, do seek alternate medical advice--as well as the advice of your current doctor. But do not abandon your prescribed medication without speaking to some physician about your condition and your concerns.

You should also note that there are definite dangers any time you stop taking any kind of pharmaceutical. We'll discuss these briefly.

IS IT POSSIBLE TO WITHDRAW FROM DRUGS?

Usually because of unpleasant side effects (like

the many examples listed below), patients may decide, on their own, to stop taking a particular medication.

In the case of hypertensive drugs, the result is usually that the patient's blood pressure increases rapidly, back to the level where it had been before the medication was prescribed. The lesson, which doctors tend to emphasize, is that patients must not take their drug treatment into their own hands.

Again, in the case of hypertensive drugs, many physicians feel that those who go on them must expect to stay on them indefinitely--meaning for the rest of their lives.

But, according to encouraging mainstream medical experiments, in some cases patients have been able to go off blood-pressure therapy completely, with no return of high blood pressure.

Here are the current guidelines of most cardiovascular professionals:

1. Don't stop taking medications unilaterally (without your doctor's advice). It can be extremely dangerous to throw all drugs inside and suffer the long-term consequences of uncontrolled high blood pressure.

2. Don't try taking a day off from your medication in order to minimize some side effect. Antihypertensive drugs are designed to be taken regularly.

3. Expect to stay on your medication for at least a year before conside ring going off it.

4. Instead of going "cold turkey," follow the "step-down" method, gradually decreasing your medication. Doctors usually recommend patients who've

been doing well reduce dosages a few milligrams at a time. If no ill effects are observed, further reductions can be discussed.

5. If you're unhappy with any drug, talk to your doctor about it. If your doctor is unresponsive, consult another doctor.

6. While following your drug regimen, also pursue non-drug treatments. In the case of high-blood pressure, it would be almost impossible to stop drug therapy without ongoing non-drug therapies to control the condition.

Nutritionists agree that the best practice is to withdraw from any medication slowly, the "step-down" method, and at the same time, increase nutrition slowly, on what we may call "reverse vectors."

A few simple rules may help: the longer an individual has been on a drug, the longer withdrawal from it should be. A range of two weeks for short-term, and six weeks for long-term, might be generally recommended, with a variety of terms between these extremes.

It is essential to know for what condition any and all drugs have been prescribed and what improvements can firmly be expected from specific nutrients. In cases of high blood pressure, a person should not consider withdrawal from a drug unless vitamin B-3, in the niacin form (not niacinamide), was being introduced, and increased just a little faster than the rate of withdrawal from the drug. (For more on niacin, see Chapter 12, "The Best Heart Medicine?")

In some cases of high cholesterol (but not the life-threatening ones), "reverse vectoring" could be set aside in favor of an immediate diet high in soluble fiber. Many other nutrients (which we'll discuss later on) should accompany this kind of changeover.

MEASURING THE RISKS OF CARDIOVAS-CULAR DRUGS

With all the above reservations, all of us definitely need to know what current medical research has learned about the potential downside from the most commonly dispensed medications for lowering cholesterol and blood pressure.

In addition to side effects, there are additional risk of what are called interactions.

Many heart patients are prescribed so many pills that they lose track. Sometimes doctors recommend several medications, believing two or more drugs will be safer or more effective than a single one. Other people have several health problem and are taking a regimen of medications for each--or are getting drugs from more than one doctor.

But drugs often have multiple actions, which can alter the effects of one another. Some interactions between cardiovascular medications may be intended--such as low doses of two blood-pressure medications that may also lower blood-pressure, with fewer side effects than a high dose of a single agent.

But often drugs interact in ways that can be extremely harmful. One might slow absorption of a second; another might accelerate its absorption.

A final pitfall: Over-the-counter medications may also interact with prescription drugs.

PREVENTING INTERACTIONS

Contemplating possible drug interactions can be very frightening--especially after you've read through some of the complications below. Many physicians, however, maintain that the use of more than one drug to treat cardiovascular disease is often essential, and claim that multiple drug therapy can be both safe and effective--provided that all potential interactions are anticipated.

They urge patients to give their doctors a complete list of all their medications each time they visit. The list should include over-the-counter preparations as well as those prescribed.

Doctors also advise that those who take prescription drugs should read the package insert, which lists drugs that can potentially interact with their medication. The dispensing pharmacist should also be consulted, if the patient has further questions.

PROBLEMS WITH ACE INHIBITORS

Angiotensin-converting enzyme (ACE) inhibitors are relatively new and are very expensive. They cost 50 to 60 cents per pill, in contrast to diuretics, which in generic form cost as little as 3 cents per pill or capsule.

ACE inhibitors cause arteries throughout the body to dilate and are among the most widely used blood-pressure-reducing agents. Because these vasodilators lower the resistance against which the heart must work, ACE inhibitors are also used for the treatment of congestive heart failure due to a weakened left ventricle. The left ventricle, one of the two lower chambers of the heart, pumps blood into the general circulation.

Examples of ACE inhibitors are captopril (Capoten), enalapril (Vasotec), and lisinopril (Zestril, Prinivil).

ACE inhibitors are frequently combined with other drugs that help people who have high blood pressure or heart failure, such as diuretics that promote loss of fluid from the body or other vasodilator drugs.

In combination with these drugs, ACE inhibitors exert an even more powerful blood-pressure-lowering effect--sometimes too powerful. Patients can develop lightheadedness or even fainting spells if their blood pressure is too low. For problems using ACE inhibitors with diuretics, see section on diuretics below.

Possible side effects: Hypertension; dizziness; weakness; loss of appetite, nausea; hacking cough; swelling (especially around the face); rashes; loss of taste.

Caution: ACE inhibitors should not be used by anyone with impaired liver function or by pregnant or breast-feeding women. Side effects may be even more severe on older people.

The ACE inhibitors can also trigger kidney failure in patients with kidney problems, and sometimes lead to a decrease in the white blood cells, a factor in bone marrow disease.

PROBLEMS WITH ANTICOAGULANTS

These drugs, which prevent blood clots from forming around damaged tissue, are useful in preventing heart attacks or strokes after heart surgery.

Examples: warfarin (Coumadin, Panwarfarin).

Possible side effects: Excessive bleeding or bruising; nausea, vomiting; hair loss.

Other cautions: As with ACE inhibitors, anticoagulants should not be taken by pregnant women or people with impaired liver function. In addition, they should be avoided by those with impaired kidney function. Generally, they are temporary measures, prescribed for 6 to 8 months following surgery or cardiovascular injury such as a stroke or heart attack.

Possible interactions: Unfortunately, the anticoagulant warfarin interacts with many kind of drugs, including aspirin, oral contraceptives and laxatives.

Several drugs slow the rate at which the body breaks down warfarin, including the cholesterol-lowering agent lovastatin (Mevacor), the antihypertensive medication methyldopa (Aldomet), and some antiarrhythmic drugs such as amiodarone hydrochloride (Cordarone), propafenone (Rhythmol), and quinidine (Quinidex).

With slower breakdown of warfarin, a patient's clotting mechanism might become dangerously impaired. The cholesterol-lowering agent cholestyramine interferes with the gastrointestinal absorption of warfarin, diminishing its effects.

The complete list of medications that can affect the actions of warfarin is quite long. People who are on a steady dose of this anticoagulant should have their bleeding times closely monitored when any of these medications is started or stopped.

Patients who take warfarin should also discuss over-the-counter medications with their physician before using them. If a person uses both warfarin and aspirin (an antiplatelet, as you'll see in the next section), the risk for bleeding complications may be excessive.

PROBLEMS WITH ANTIPLATELETS

These drugs act on platelet blood cells, making them less sticky and thus less likely to clump together and form clots.

(Platelets are small blood cells essential for clotting.) For those suffering atherosclerosis, with a high risk of heart attack and stroke, antiplatelets are often prescribed as preventatives.

Examples: acetylsalicylic acid or aspirin (Alka-Seltzer, Anacin, Bayer, Bufferin, Ecotrin), dipyridamole (Persantine).

Possible side effects: Nausea, vomiting, indigestion.

Other cautions: Aspirin in low doses is the most common antiplatelet drug prescribed. Antiplatelets also reduce angina both in severity and frequency. Those with digestive system problems such as ulcers or bleeding disorders should only take platelets with extreme caution. The same goes for breast-feeding or pregnant women.

Note: Antioxidant vitamins can also act as anti-platelets--and without side effects. See "Antioxidants and Heart Surgery" in Chapter Three.

PROBLEMS WITH BETA BLOCKERS

For high blood pressure, the drugs of first choice are usually beta blockers (which reduce heart rate and blood output) along with diuretics.

Beta blockers work by blocking the action of certain receptors (beta receptors) in the heart, blood vessels and other parts of the body, which would otherwise increase the heart rate.

These drugs are frequently used for several cardiovascular conditions, including high blood pressure, heart-rhythm abnormalities (arrhythmias) and angina (the chest pain or discomfort that indicates an insufficient blood supply to the heart muscle). In addition, this class of drugs is routinely prescribed for people who have had heart attacks. Some examples of beta blockers are atenolol (Tenormin), propranolol (Inderal), nadolol (Corgard) and metoprolol (Lopressor).

Problems: Beta blockers tend to cause spasm in the bronchial tubes, so they are definitely not indicated for people with asthma. They are also not recommended for those with circulatory problems in their hands and feet.

Possible side effects: Nausea; insomnia; nightmares; impotence; lethargy and weakness; depression; cold hands and feet due to reduced circulation; excessively slow heart rate; elevated triglyceride counts; declines in HDL cholesterol; and worsening of angina pectoris pains.

Possible dangerous interactions: Since Beta blockers slow the heart rate, if a patient uses another medication that has the same effect, the interaction of the two drugs can produce unwanted consequences. Verapamil (Calan, Isoptin) and diltiazem (Cardizem, Dilacor) are two calcium-channel blocking agents that slow the heart and are also frequently used for many of the same conditions as beta blockers. The combination of a beta blocker and these calcium blockers can make the heart rate of some people decline to 40-50 beats per minute (sometimes even slower) and may even cause the person to become dizzy or lose consciousness because too little blood is being pumped to the brain.

Beta blockers and calcium-channel blockers can interact in other ways. Since both drugs decrease the forcefulness of the heart's contractions, some people can develop heart failure when these medications are used together--even if the heart rate is in the normal range.

Beta blockers also can pose problems for people with diabetes, particularly for those who take insulin to lower blood-sugar levels. If these patients use too much insulin, their blood-sugar levels decline to a dangerously low point.

Ordinarily, the body responds with sweating and a rapid heart rate that can alert the patient to the low sugar level. However, the presence of a beta blocker can block the symptoms that come from low blood sugar and prevent the patient from recognizing the insulin reaction. Therefore, people with diabetes who take beta blockers must recognize all the signs of low blood sugar, including weakness.

PROBLEMS WITH CALCIUM-CHANNEL BLOCKERS

Calcium-channel blockers are relatively new drugs. Verapamil (Calan, Isoptin), diltiazem (Cardizem, Dilacor) and nifedipine (Procardia, Adalat) are commonly used to treat high blood pressure and angina. Verapamil and diltiazem may be given for arrhythmias and to decrease the heart rate. Doctors may explain to a patient that these medications will help relax blood vessels, slow heart rate and lower blood pressure.

So what are the problems? For starters, physicians need to warn patients that even a slightly increased dosage can cause a dangerous droop in blood pressure and put them in the hospital.

They should further explain that the addition of calcium-channel blockers to other blood-pressure-lowering medications can also lead to symptoms of low blood pressure, including dizziness.

And when beta blockers (see below) are combined with verapamil or diltiazem, excessive slowing of the heart can result. These two calcium-channel blockers can also cause a slow heart rate if combined with digoxin, another medication commonly used by heart patients. Verapamil and diltiazem can also raise the level of digoxin in the bloodstream.

All calcium blockers may cause headaches, dizziness and flushing.

Far more serious:

In September, 1995, there were dramatic stories about one calcium channel blocker for high blood pressure being linked to heart attack. The drug was nifedipine--specifically a variety of nifedipine known as "immediate-release" drug, which can cause extreme effects on blood pressure. (Sustained-release, calcium channel blockers try to avoid sharp effects.)

To reassure many panicky people, the American Heart Association (AHA) issued a quick press release, which estimated that if 1,000 patients take the particular calcium channel blocker, 16 may have a heart attack. Taking either of the other two main classes--a diuretic drug or beta blocker--10 would have a heart attack.

Do you find this reassuring?

Predictably the U.S. Food and Drug Administration (FDA) also issued a statement in support of calcium channel blockers.

PROBLEMS WITH DIURETICS

Diuretics are often called water pills, since they reduce the volume of the body's blood and fluids by increasing the kidney's elimination of sodium and water. (For this same reason, they are sometimes referred to as "volume reducers.")

How much fluid do they cause to be eliminated? Usually about two-quarts. This lessening of fluid levels also reduces both heart action and pressure on the walls of blood vessels.

On the positive side, diuretics are the only blood pressure drugs proven to decrease the incidence of strokes and heart failure.

Examples: chlorthalidone (Hygroton), hydrochlorothiazide (Esidrix, Hydro-Diuril, Oretic), metolazone (Diulo, Mykrox, Zaroxolyn), bumetanide

(Bumex), furosemide (Lasix), amiloride (Midamore), spironolactone (Aldactone).

"Water pills" such as hydrochlorothiazide or furosemide (Lasix) promote urination and removal of excess fluid from the body. Unfortunately, water is not the only substance lost from the body because of these medications. Potassium and magnesium leave with the urine, and low blood levels of these chemicals can cause life-threatening heart-rhythm abnormalities, since potassium is essential for proper muscle function.

The danger of low potassium or magnesium levels is especially critical for people who use digoxin. This medication can cause heart-rhythm abnormalities--particularly if blood levels of potassium or magnesium are low. Therefore, those who take diuretics and digoxin should undergo regular blood tests (approximately every six months) to ensure body chemicals are in the normal range. Abnormal results should be corrected through the use of potassium or magnesium supplements; dietary changes may help as well.

Other side effects: Some diuretics cause blood-sugar levels (and sometimes cholesterol levels) to rise. For people with a tendency toward diabetes, this may cause the blood-sugar level to rise high enough to cause symptoms. It can also lead to glucose intolerance, an inability of the body to metabolize, use and store sugar, as in diabetes mellitus.

For those already under treatment for diabetes with insulin or pills, dosages often must be increased if diuretics are prescribed. A patient already taking medication for an extremely high cholesterol level may also need to have the dose adjusted.

In other patients, diuretics can cause overproduction of uric acid, which can trigger an attack of gout.

Even more possible side effects: Lethargy; cramps; rash; impotence.

Possible interactions: Since diuretics often cause potassium levels in the blood to fall, it may seem beneficial that ACE inhibitors tend to cause a mild increase in the blood-potassium level. But the addition of ACE inhibitors can cause trouble for people who use potassium supplements with their diuretics, or who use other medications to increase potassium levels, such as commonly used salt substitutes or nonsteroidal anti-inflammatory agents such as ibuprofen or naproxyn. With two drugs acting to raise potassium levels, the body's natural mechanisms for controlling potassium can be overwhelmed, and potassium may soar to dangerous levels. Blood tests to monitor potassium levels after the addition of ACE inhibitors can prevent such complications.

PROBLEMS WITH LIPID-LOWERING DRUGS

Lipids, as we've discussed, are simply fats circulating in the blood. By reducing these blood fats, the likelihood of atherosclerosis can also be reduced or altogether prevented.

There are two principal kinds of lipid-lowering medications:

(1) those that act on the liver by blocking the conversion of fatty acids to lipids; and

(2) those that act to reduce the absorption of bile

salts (substances containing large amounts of cholesterol that are secreted from the liver into the intestine) into the blood.

Examples: cholestyramine (Questran, Questran Light), colestipol (Colestid), gemfibrozil (Lopid), lovastatin (Mevacor), probucol (Lorelco).

Cholestyramine (Questran) and colestipol (Colestid) are sand-like materials which bind bile salts in the intestine and allow fat and cholesterol to be eliminated in the stool. Unfortunately, cholestyramine can do exactly the same thing with many cardiac medications, including warfarin, metoprolol, and digoxin. These and all other medicines should be taken at least one hour before or four hours after taking cholestyramine, and drug levels should be closely followed.

With cholestyramine and colestipol, cholesterol can be reduced by 20%, but triglyceride levels may increase in certain patients--for example, those who already have elevated levels of these blood fats, people with diabetes (whether or not they are taking insulin), or women taking estrogen supplements. They can have the side effects of bloating, nausea, indigestion and constipation, and also interfere with the absorption of many other drugs from the stomach and intestine.

Gemfibrozil (Lopid) has a limited effect in lowering cholesterol levels, but significantly lowers triglyceride levels (40% decrease on average), while raising HDL cholesterol by 20%. While negative side effects are not common, abnormal liver tests or gallstone formation have been known to occur.

Gemfibrozil, lovastatin and clofibrate can increase the risk of bleeding in patients taking warfarin, and most patients will need to reduce their warfarin dose when these drugs are added. Gemfibrozil taken in combination with lovastatin, pravastatin or simvastatin can sometimes lead to severe muscle, liver and kidney damage. The U.S. Food and Drug Administration recommends against these combinations.

Lovastatin (Mevacor), one of a drug class known as "statins," lowers total cholesterol by 25%, decreases LDL cholesterol by 35% and increases HDL cholesterol by 10% on average. (These encouraging statistics are from three major studies, which monitored more than 15,000 people for five yeras.) It is usually well tolerated, but a temporary increase in liver enzyme tests is seen in 2-3% of patients, so periodic blood liver enzyme tests are recommended.

Mevacor, made by Merck & Co., is one of the two largest-selling cholesterol-lowering drugs. But it is priced out of reach of many American consumers--$15 to $40 a week to take recommended dosages.

Probucol (Lorelco) is an antioxidant which lowers cholesterol by about 15%, but is associated with a decrease in HDL level by similar, if not greater amounts.

Often, when single drug therapy is found inadequate to lower cholesterol levels, more than one cholesterol-lowering medication is used in combination. Examples of such drug combinations include either cholestyramine or colestid along with niacin (nicotinic acid, vitamin B-3), gemfibrozil or a "statin" drug.

PROBLEMS WITH NITRATES

Nitrates relax the muscles surrounding the blood vessels, causing them to widen (or dilate), which improves blood flow through the heart. For this reason, nitrates are the oldest coronary artery medication, especially used to treat angina pectoris. They are also used for people with heart failure, because the vasodilating effects decrease work for the heart and ease congestion caused by fluid in the lungs.

Examples: nitroglycerin (Deponit NTG, Minitran, Nitro-Bid, Nitrogard, Nitroglyn, Nitrol, Nitrolingual, Nitrong, Nitrostat, Transderm-Nitro, Tridil), isosorbide dinitrate (Dilatrate-SR, Iso-Bid, Isordil, Sorbitrate, Sorbitrate SA).

Possible interactions: The dilation of blood vessels induced by nitrates causes a drop in blood pressure, and this drop can be accentuated in people who are using other medications that lower blood pressure, including diuretics, ACE inhibitors and beta blockers.

Nitrates also cause an increase in heart rate as the body tries to compensate for the lowered blood pressure. Therefore, patients who are also taking other blood-pressure-reducing drugs may feel their heart race. Patients on nifedipine may even have a worsening of angina because of the increase in heart rate.

PROBLEMS WITH DIGOXIN

Digoxin is prescribed to treat congestive heart failure and to control the heart rate in atrial fibrillation, a condition characterized by rapid irregular beats of the heart's upper chambers. Because high digoxin doses can actually poison the heart and other organs, dosage must be carefully measured to achieve a blood concentration neither too low, which would be ineffective, nor too high.

Unfortunately, many cardiovascular drugs raise or lower levels of digoxin in the bloodstream, while others change the sensitivity of the heart to digoxin's actions. Among medications that raise blood levels of digoxin are calcium-channel blockers such as verapamil and some antiarrhythmic medicines such as quinidine (Quinidex), amiodarone (Cordarone), and propafenone (Rhythmol).

During addition or discontinuation of these medications, digoxin levels must be carefully monitored and the dose of digoxin reduced. Other medications, including resins such as the cholesterol-lowering agent cholestyramine (Questran), decrease digoxin levels by interfering with gastrointestinal absorption.

GETTING THE BEST OF MEDICAL TECHNOLOGY

It's a scary list of side effects, isn't it? And in subsequent chapters we're going to present dozens and dozens of drug-free ways to lower cholesterol and blood pressure.

But let us repeat: These cardiovascular medications, for all their strange names and possible complications, have saved many lives and will save many more--pehaps yours.

And there are many other wonders of medical science, which, if used properly, can help diagnose and treat heart disease. The following chapter offers a quick survey at the latest innovations in cardio-medical technology.

III. BENEFITS OF MEDICAL TECHNOLOGY

GIVE MEDICAL TECHNOLOGY ITS DUE

While the emphasis of this book is on natural remedies for heart-related illness, it would be wrong not to applaud the advances made in combatting coronary disease by standard medical science, especially in the last thirty years. These advances--in diagnostic methods, surgical techniques and drugs--have saved and prolonged millions of lives.

Unfortunately, these breakthroughs have contributed little in the way of prevention. Coronary disease continues to occur at alarming rates, creating hordes of fresh candidates for more advanced medical intervention. Doctors may talk about prevention and wellness, but their focus remains on treating illness.

Doctors, of course, also have a way of sounding cock-sure of their diagnosis and advice. In previous generations the patient was expected to accept the doctor's pronouncements--without understanding or questioning. In the opinion of many, that was a passive role that treated the medical consumer as a child.

These days, we're happy to say, more and more of us are asking hard questions of our doctors. We are becoming savvy medical consumers. As part of that, we are beginning to take responsibility for our own health and health-care.

Which is why it's useful to inform yourself about current medical theory and practice on coronary disease--today's methods for diagnosis, treatment and surgical intervention. Perhaps you will never have to consider the options discussed below, but someone you know probably will--a friend, a colleague, a loved one. You should therefore learn the basics.

And it would be a grievous oversight to launch into the wonderful world of alternative treatments (which we'll do next chapter) without giving modern medical science its due.

THE DIAGNOSTICIAN'S TOOLKIT

Medical specialists have an amazing array of tools to pinpoint heart problems. These range from standard physical exams to sophisticated nuclear medical techniques. The purpose of all of these is to ascertain the extent of damage to the heart muscle or the risk of future damage.

On the basis of these tests, a doctor may prescribe heart medication, continue current medication or recommend medical treatment. In some cases the doctor will recommend corrective surgery or angioplasty (balloon dilation). If the condition is less threatening, the doctor may simply outline corrective lifestyle changes.

COMPUTER BLOOD PRESSURE MONITORS

Sitting at a computer keyboard endless hours is, to put it mildly, hazardous to your health. Typing and moving a mouse does little for cardiovascular fitness.

But some new PC software and hardware may help your health, by monitoring and controlling your blood pressure.

Dynapulse 200M (Pulse Metric, [800] 927-8573) is a device that plugs into the serial port of a PC or Mac to measure and record blood pressure and pulse rate.

The Dynapulse, like the home blood pressure kit, comes with a cuff that temporarily restricts blood flow in your upper arm. But instead of listening through a stethoscope, the device measures blood pressure and pulse and sends the data to the screen. You can save the data to a disk and view a line chart on how you're doing over time.

Admittedly, the Dynapulse, with a suggested retail price of $179 and a discounted price of about $120, is a bit expensive. To save money, use a manual blood pressure gauge and a spreadsheet program to keep track of the numbers. For around $30 you can buy a portable home sphygmomanometer, which, if used properly, is very accurate.

LOWERING CHOLESTEROL VIA COMPUTER

Patients who had regular telephone consultations with a computer lowered their cholesterol, exercised more and did better at taking their medicine, according to one researcher who predicts the approach will become a major way of delivering health care.

The results came from three experiments in which patients called a talking computer that assessed their conditions and progress, and offered custom-made guidance through recorded messages.

Patients like the approach, and it's only a dollar or two per call, said Dr. Robert Friedman, chief of the Medical Information Systems Unit at the Boston University Medical Center.

It might be able to save money when used to monitor people with chronic diseases like diabetes, by keeping them out of the hospital, he said.

Computer-controlled phone conversations "will be a major means of delivering health care in the 21st century," he said.

Friedman described the experiments at the 1996 annual meeting of the American Psychological Association.

Participants talked to the computer by pressing numbers on a push-button phone. Researchers are working on ways to let callers just talk instead.

One study involved 68 sedentary elderly people in the Boston area. To see if the computer chats could get them to walk for exercise, they were randomly assigned to have either a weekly call along with their usual care from their doctors, or just their usual care.

As with the other experiments, each participant was expected to make the call. But if he or she missed the arranged time, the computer called instead.

In the conversations, the computer helped patients overcome obstacles to exercise, such as not knowing where to walk or how to make it fun. For example, it suggested getting a friend to come along.

Once the person began walking, the computer tracked his or her progress toward the goal of walking 60 minutes a week and offered encouragement.

After three months, those who had the computer conversations walked an average of 34 minutes a day, vs. 21 minutes for those in the comparison group.

In a different study, 65 adults with high cholesterol were randomly assigned to call the computer twice a week along with getting their usual medical care, or to get only their usual care.

The computer quizzed them on what they ate and how much. Then they got tailored guidance on improving their diets.

At the end of three months, those who had chatted with the computer showed an average 17-point drop in their cholesterol levels, compared with three points for the other participants.

The third experiment involved 267 elderly people who were taking medication for high blood pressure. The goal was to help them take their pills as prescribed.

The computer asked how often each participant had missed a dose, explored the reasons and offered tips for overcoming the problem. In later conversations, it asked whether the tips worked. If not, it offered new tips.

Overall, compliance improved by 18 percent in the computer group and 12 percent in the others. The computer users also showed a bigger drop in blood pressure.

Wayne Velicer of the University of Rhode Island, who is studying the use of computers to help people quit smoking, said Friedman's results show "tremendous promise."

BASIC CHOLESTEROL TESTING

Medical professionals recommend that people over the age of 20 have their blood cholesterol level tested every 5 years. The National Cholesterol Education Program (NCEP) classifies total blood cholesterol levels as:

Desirable (less than 200)

Borderline (200-239)

High (greater than or equal to 240)

Other physicians go farther. They suggest that everyone, regardless of age, have an annual blood cholesterol test.

Fact is, most Americans don't know their blood cholesterol level. Some are discouraged from doing so by the cost of lab tests, which can run $50 (though they are usually covered by health insurance). Others are too busy, or perhaps too lazy, to schedule an office visit.

These days, one convenient alternative to the doctor or lab test is the home cholesterol test. Technical advances have made it feasible to perform this measurement with only a drop of blood instead of a tube-ful. The question is, how reliable are these tests?

HOME CHOLESTEROL TESTING, PROS & CONS

Cholesterol kits have been available for years in Europe, but approved by the U.S. government for home use only in 1994. For around $20 you can buy a single-use, disposable plastic "cassette" to hold the blood, a "lancet" to prick a finger, a gauze pad and written instructions on how to interpret the test results. Also included is a toll-free "Help Line" number for customers to call the manufacturer (Johnson & Johnson) with questions. Instead of waiting a couple of days for results, you can get them in a little more than a quarter-hour.

* How It Works:

The patient pricks a finger with the lancet and places a few blood droplets in a well in the plastic cassette, where the blood is filtered to remove some of the cells. The remaining blood is then exposed to enzymes that separate cholesterol into various parts. As these spread along a treated chemical wick, a purple dye moves as well: the more cholesterol in the blood, the farther the chemical will travel. After about 20 minutes, a reading is made based on how far the purple color has moved.

The consensus of medical opinion seems to be that, if used properly, these tests give an accurate reading 97 percent of the time--a terrific score. In lab testing, results from finger-stick tests vary by only about 5% from values obtained with standard hospital equipment.

WARNINGS ABOUT HOME CHOLES-TEROL TESTING

Despite the amazingly high accuracy of these tests when properly given and interpreted, there are problems associated with them:

1. Users are warned that failure to follow instructions can lead to false readings. Mistakes can result from using too little blood, by waiting too long or not long enough, or by running the test in direct sunlight. Also: Even a single dose of Tylenol or vitamin C can skew the results.

2. Interpretation of the final color-change reading may be ambiguous.

3. Home tests should never be attempted by hemophiliacs or anyone who takes blood-thinning medicine, due to the danger of excessive bleeding.

4. Cholesterol levels in everyone vary from day to day. Thus, measures of cholesterol at two different times might vary by several points (mg/dl) in the absence of any meaningful change. There is, for instance, no value in testing them after a rich meal or a week of dieting.

5. People with a truly elevated cholesterol level may get a falsely low result on a home test--and therefore not seek medical attention or make healthy lifestyle changes. On the other hand, false high results could lead to unnecessary anxiety. Even with correct readings, patients may not be able to evaluate whether a change is important.

6. Another disadvantage of the home finger-stick test is that it doesn't give a complete lipid profile, only

the total blood-cholesterol level, without breaking down the lipid into the "good" high-density lipoprotein (HDL) cholesterol, which is associated with a decreased risk for heart attack, and the "bad" low-density lipoprotein (LDL) cholesterol, which carries an increased heart-attack risk.

7. For all these reasons, home tests are not designed to replace an annual checkup, including cholesterol reading, with your doctor. They are useful, however, for those with high or borderline cholesterol levels who want to monitor themselves between doctor visits, much as some people with hypertension use home blood-pressure monitors to work with their physicians. Others at increased risk of heart disease should ask their doctor about home testing.

ELECTROCARDIOGRAM OR ECG

The ECG measures your heart's electrical activity. It can be performed while you're resting or exercising. But at rest, the heart's oxygen needs aren't that great, so the heart may be able to compensate for any slowdowns due to clogged coronary arteries. This is why an exercise stress test reveal a great deal more to the doctor. It can be useful in diagnosing heart problems and in prescribing safe and effective exercise programs.

In the exercise lab a nurse or technician applies electrodes to various points on the front of the upper body, sometimes on the back. Generally, ten or more electrodes are needed to allow the heart's electrical activity to be monitored from various directions.

The electrodes are connected to a series of wires hooked up to an electrocardiograph machine.

Exercise stress tests are most commonly performed on treadmills and divided into several stages, each more challenging. The doctor stops the test when the patient achieves a preset maximal heart rate, when abnormal symptoms are noted, or if you complain of pain or serious fatigue.

How safe are exercise stress tests? Quite safe, even for people with cardiovascular disease.

The American Heart Association recommends an exercise stress test under the following conditions:

1. If you're a sedentary, over 40 and going to participate in a vigorous exercise program.

2. If you're under 40 and have risk factors or a strong family history of coronary heart disease.

3. At any age, if you have cardiovascular disease or its symptoms.

ELECTRON BEAM SCANNERS

Cardiology re-searchers say that a new generation of noninvasive, predictive tests are available via a new type of scanning machine, known as an ultrafast CT or electron beam CT. These offer tests, including heart scans, that can see the incipient (or beginning) growth of artery-clogging plaque.

The new machines take X-ray images of the heart so rapidly that they can snap the exposures between beats, avoiding the fuzziness that can occur with normal CT scans. A diagnostic radiologist at the Mayo Clinic in Rochester, MN., explained that the ultrafast CTs take pictures in a tenth of a second, while a conventional CT scanner require about 2 seconds-- during which time the heart beats twice.

Ultrafast CT scanners can't show actual plaque, but they can show flecks of calcium in coronary arteries. These appear as bright white flakes on the dark-gray X-ray pictures. By detecting these calcium deposits, ultrafast CT scans seem to isolate atherosclerosis long before it has had a chance to advance.

Other advantages to Ultrafast CT:

* Radiation exposure is less than for a regular CT scan.

* Painless, non-invasive.

* Convenient: No fasting, dieting or other preparation necessary. The actual scan takes only about ten minutes.

For more information: An Los Angeles-area provider of these scans, along with a detailed risk factor assessment, located at the UCLA Medical Center, may be able to recommend a facility in your area. Call HealthPro Heart Workup, 800-408-SCAN.

NUCLEAR MEDICINE

These techniques offer cardiologists a way to look inside your heart to determine its condition and to recommend the proper treatment.

* Radionuclide Ventriculography.

In this test, a tiny amount of radioactive isotope is injected into the bloodstream. These isotopes decay so quickly that they remain in the body only long enough for the test to be completed.

When the radioactive material passes through the heart, the doctor can accurately measure the percentage of blood the left ventricle ejects during contraction--and thus determine if there is severe left ventricle dysfunction, which shows high risk for future heart problems.

* Thallium Scan.

This techniques can improve upon the accuracy of an exercise test. It's commonly employed after a heart attack to measure the extent of heart damage.

Toward the end of an exercise test, the patient is injected with thallium-201, a radioactive isotope, through an intravenous line. It allows doctors to see the parts of the heart where the blood supply is inadequate because the thallium won't reach those areas. The doctor can also see where a heart attack occurred.

Three or four hours after the exercise test, the thallium is remeasured. This distinguishes areas of temporary blockage from areas permanently damaged during the heart attack. Thallium will remain only in the damaged part of the heart.

* Echocardiography. This ultrasound procedure bounces sound waves off the heart's surface. The results are converted into pictures the cardiologist can read.

* Holter Monitoring. This procedure is used when the doctor suspects left-ventricular dysfunction. It helps detect frequent irregular heartbeats or "PVCs" (premature ventricular contractions).

With Holter monitoring, the patient wears a small tape recorder for at least 24 hours, usually on a belt around the waist. This monitor records the heart's electrical signals. They can be played back using special equipment that helps single out those fleeting heart rhythm disturbances not captured during an ordinary ECG.

* Angiogram or Angiography. Angiography helps determine if specialized heart surgery is needed. A coronary angiogram locates the actual sites of narrowing in coronary arteries and traces a map for any subsequent surgery.

The angiogram is performed in what is called a cardiac catheterization laboratory ("cath lab"). The patient lies on a table under an X-ray camera, hooked up to an ECG monitor. The area where the catheter will be inserted is shaved, cleaned and anesthetized.

The cardiologist inserts a thin plastic tube into an artery in the groin or arm, gradually moving the catheter up to the arteries in the heart. Dye is injected into the coronary arteries while an X-ray machine takes rapid exposures. Next, the catheter is moved inside the left ventricle, where dye is also injected. As the physician views what's happening on the TV monitor, the X-rays are being recorded on a videocassette.

Coronary angiography is extremely safe. Performed correctly, the death rate is less than 0.2 percent and the risk of heart attack, stroke or severe bleeding less than 0.5 percent.

WHEN BLOOD VESSEL 'REPAIRS' ARE NECESSARY

Evaluating diagnostic procedures--stress tests, angiograms and left ventriculography and other pertinent information--doctors decide whether a patient might benefit from an angioplasty or coronary artery bypass surgery.

Both these procedures are designed to reestablish an adequate blood supply to areas of the heart deprived because of blockages in the coronary arteries. An angioplasty achieves the goal by widening the arteries at the sites where they've become narrowed by plaque. Bypass surgery achieves the same results by detouring the blood around the narrowed parts of the coronary arteries.

HOW ANGIOPLASTY WORKS

Every year in the U.S., nearly 400,000 angioplasties are performed with a success rate around 90%. In a small percentage of cases, however, the dilated coronary artery will become obstructed again within about six months and the procedure may need to be repeated.

Contrasted with bypass surgery, angioplasty is much less radical, requires a shorter hospital stay, costs less and has fewer complications.

As with an angiogram, angioplasty is done in the cath lab with the patient fully awake. A catheter is inserted through the arm or groin and guided into the coronary artery under X-ray monitoring.

A second catheter is then passed inside the first into the coronary artery. At the end of this second catheter is a small, deflated balloon. The cardiologist injects dye into the artery to help steer the balloon-tipped catheter into the narrowed areas. The doctor inflates the balloon within each of the blocked areas to open up the coronary artery. After the balloon is deflated, an angiogram is done to measure if the angioplasty has done its job.

Complications are rare with angioplasty, though emergency coronary bypass surgery is required in around 5% of angioplasty patients.

CORONARY ARTERY BYPASS

There are arguments pro and con concerning long-term benefits of bypass surgery. Most physicians, however, do agree that bypass surgery does prolong life.

The aim of bypass surgery is to reroute blood around a blocked coronary artery. Thereafter, increased blood flow should eliminate the chest pain (angina pectoris) that occurs with exercise. Other benefits include a reduction in fatigue and medication and a restoration of well-being.

Coronary artery bypass surgery is an open-heart operation. It entails removing part of an artery or vein from one part of the body and sewing (or grafting) it onto the heart's arteries. Usually the surgeon uses one of two blood vessels as grafts--a superficial vein that runs down the inside of the leg or one of the vessels down the right and left side of the chest alongside the breast bone.

These arteries or veins are surgically connected to the coronary arteries on the surface of the heart. The connections are made in front of and behind the blockages. This way, blood flows through them, bypassing the narrowed or closed points.

ANTIOXIDANTS AND HEART SURGERY

There is growing evidence that antioxidant supplementation can help prevent free-radical damage that occurs during open- heart surgery. (For a detailed discussion of "free radicals," see "Free Radicals and Heart Disease," Chapter Four.)

The damage is caused when, in order to reduce bleeding, blood flow is purposely diverted from the heart muscle during open heart surgery. This diversion triggers a surge of free-radical production in heart tissue, which can cause tremendous structural damage.

In one study, five days before undergoing coronary artery bypass surgery, a number of patients were given 100,000 IU of vitamin A and 400 IU of vitamin E daily, while another group was given no such supplementation.

Biopsy samples were taken of heart tissue before diverting blood away from the heart and after blood flow was restored. Results showed a decrease in free-radicals in samples of those who took antioxidants, but an increase in those who took no antioxidants.

The evidence certainly justifies a person facing such surgery requesting that antioxidant supplementation be given in advance. If surgeons are not responsive, of course, antioxidants require no prescription. The patient can supplement himself or herself, and thus help protect the heart during the upcoming trauma.

BYPASS A BYPASS WITH CHELATION THERAPY?

The late Dr. Linus Pauling advanced the idea that EDTA chelation therapy could accomplish the same thing as a bypass operation--at a fraction of the cost and risk.

EDTA (ethylene diaminetetra-acetic acid) is not a vitamin, but a synthetic amino acid available by prescription. This protein-like material, injected intravenously, ties up or "chelates" minerals in the bloodstream. Numerous tests, cited by Pauling, Dr. Morton Walker, Dr. Sidney Alexander and others, have shown that injections of EDTA can help pull calcium from atherosclerotic plaque from arteries. Blood pressure becomes normal and circulatory improvement takes place throughout the blood system.

Orthodox physicians, however, rarely recommend chelation therapy, and rarely even mention it in informing patients of the different therapies available to them.

HEART VALVE SURGERY

A human heart beats more than 100,000 times each day. So its valves must flex, stretch and hold back pressure hundreds of millions of times in an average lifetime.

You have four heart valves. Several things can cause problems:

* A heart valve may not be normal at birth and require immediate repair.

* A minor birth defect may cause problems later in life.

* Diseases such as rheumatic fever or bacterial infections may cause scarring or damages.

* The aging process may weaken or harden the valve.

Any heart valve problems greatly increases the heart's work, which may cause the heart to enlarge. When the heart can no longer enlarge, heart failure soon follows.

Some with diseased heart valves can get by with careful medical supervision. Others may need surgery to repair or replace the valve.

Several types of replacement valve mechanisms are used. Biological tissue valves use animal valves or the aortic valve from a human donor.

Mechanical valves are artificial devices made of durable metals. They're longer-lasting than tissue valves, but, as they aren't natural to the body, they may cause blood clots to form. To prevent this, people with mechanical valves must take medication every day for the rest of their lives.

Caution: Those with heart valve problems need to inform their dentist and other doctors so antibiotics can be prescribed before and after procedures likely to cause bleeding. Otherwise, bacteria could release into the bloodstream during these procedures and cause an infection in the heart called bacterial endocarditis.

Doctors and dentists also need to know if a patient is taking anticoagulant medications so they can make adjustments to prevent excessive bleeding.

WHAT MAKES PACEMAKERS TICK?

Artificial pacemakers are science's solution to the electrical problem of a slow heartbeat.

Actually your heart has a natural pacemaker, which triggers electrical impulses that cause the muscle to contract and pump blood. Impulses travel from the pacemaker cells down certain electrical paths in the muscle walls. So long as these impulses occur at regular intervals, your heart beats at a rhythmic pace.

Problems, however, can alter your heart's rhythm. Your heartbeat may be slow and often irregular. Or it may sometimes be normal and sometimes too fast or too slow. In either case blood isn't being pumped efficiently. An artificial pacemaker is designed to make your heart beat more regularly so that enough oxygen and nourishment can get to your body's cells.

*How they work: Pacemaker systems have two parts: a small battery-powered unit producing the electrical impulses that start the heartbeat. The generator is implanted beneath the skin through a small incision. Tiny wires, implanted at the same time, connecting the generator to the heart. Impulses flow through these wires to the heart and are timed to slow at regular intervals just as impulses from the heart's natural pacemaker normally do.

"Demand pacemakers" are designed to work only when needed. A sensing device shuts off the pacemaker if the heart beats faster than a certain rate. When beats are slower than the pacemaker rate, the sensing device turns the pacemaker on again, something like a thermostat.

Having a pacemaker implanted is a relatively simple procedure, not nearly as invasive as coronary bypass or heart valve surgery. The procedure usually requires a short stay in the hospital. By current estimates, more than 130,000 U.S. patients annually have pacemakers implanted to regulate their heartbeats.

Caution: Medical researchers warn those dependent on cardiac pacemakers to avoid using digital cellular telephones because of the potential for hazardous interference. Clinical trials have confirmed previous evidence that digital telephones emit signals that can cause pacemakers to speed up or temporarily shut off. Interference is most common when the phones were held over the chest. (Interference from the older, analog cellular telephones was rare. And there is no evidence that pacemaker patients can be affected by telephones being used nearby.)

SURGICALLY IMPLANTED DEFIBRILLA-TORS

In May of 1996 the Food and Drug Administration approved expanded use of an implant device that sends electrical jolts to an ailing heart.

The surgically implanted defibrillator was designed for patients at high risk of sudden cardiac death because of abnormal rapid heart beats, as well at those who had at least one cardiac arrest and whose irregular heartbeat resisted treatment with drugs.

These defibrillators, about the size of a cassette tape, are implanted in the abdomen and connected by wires to the heart. The device is programmed to send small pacing signals to restore proper rhythm to the heart if the beat becomes irregular.

Should the pacing signal fail to correct the beat, stronger electrical shocks are sent--similar to the electrical shock paddles used by emergency room physicians to restore heartbeat.

WHAT ABOUT HEART TRANSPLANTS?

When a heart appears damaged beyond repair, so that lesser treatments won't relieve symptoms or prolong life, cardiologists may recommend a heart transplant.

This usually involves removal of the diseased heart and replacement with a healthy human heart. "Usually" because, in certain cases, the diseased heart may remain, with a healthy heart placed next to it as a booster pump.

In the early years of these revolutionary surgeries, the patient's body often rejected the new heart. Now, thanks to an increased understanding of the immune system, survival rates of heart transplants have gradually improved. Doctors now can detect early rejection long before the patient feels anything. Although antirejection drugs must be continued for life, the dose may be reduced six to eight months after the transplant.

Today, almost 2,000 Americans have heart transplants every year in more than 150 transplant centers. The current results are encouraging:

* Four out of five patients are expected to survive one year.

* Seven of ten will survive five years after their operation.

* Almost half of those who receive a transplant today will survive more than ten years.

* The longest survivors are alive more than twenty years after their transplant.

Heart transplants are only recommended for those with a high risk of dying from heart disease within a year or two.

Once a transplant patient has survived a year, the major threat comes from blockages that develop in the arteries of the transplanted heart. If abnormalities develop in how the heart muscle works or irregular heart rhythms occur, a second transplant operation may be considered.

WHAT CAN YOU DO FOR YOUR HEART?

Now that we've surveyed what physicians and medical science and technology can do for your heart, let's take a look at what you can do for it.

And we think you'll agree with us, that you--properly informed and motivated to heal yourself--can work miracles.

Notes:

_____

_____

_____

_____

_____

_____

_____

_____

IV. YOUR HEART:
THE PERPETUAL MOTION
MACHINE

FEDERAL DIETARY GUIDELINES--DO THEY WORK?

Over the years, the U.S. Department of Agriculture (USDA) has brought us the Dietary Guidelines for Americans as well as the now famous Food Guide Pyramid. If we all paid very close attention to just these two documents, it has been said by the medical establishment, we would almost certainly reduce our risk of cardiovascular disease, diabetes and certain forms of cancer.

Of course, either the guidelines don't work, or nobody's listening, or both.

YOUR HEART'S OPTIMUM LIFESPAN

We said an audacious thing at the beginning of chapter one--that we (and many researchers) believe that your heart is designed to last for about a 120 to 140 years (or twice the average human life-span)!

This is not wild speculation (though we will indulge in a little bit of wholesome speculation in this chapter).

Indeed, the heart can live and pulse vigorously outside the body, disconnected. The death of the person does not necessarily spell the death of the heart. Countless records of human sacrifices among primitive tribes and public executions among "savage" and "civilized" nations over many centuries confirm an astounding fact: the chest can be chopped open--even after a hanged victim has stopped breathing--and the heart, still alive, can literally be pulled out. It will not stop beating, even when ruthlessly yanked free from its tangle of arteries and veins.

Pulsing hearts, gripped in gore-smeared fists, have been shown to awed and staring crowds in barbaric Aztec sacrifices and at proper London executions.

Quickly, of course, the disembodied organ expends its internal energy, succumbs to exposure and starvation and expires.

But the heart appears to be empowered to outlive us. Heart tissue has been shown to live on--outside the body--almost indefinitely when given proper care.

So why should it die before its time? Or why, or how, do we interfere with its natural readiness and strength, its virtual indestructibility?

Why, indeed, do we kill it?

THE AMAZING EXPERIMENTS OF ALEXIS CARREL

Consider the research of Alexis Carrel, a Nobel Prize-winning French surgeon and biologist who died in 1944. Dr. Carrel kept tissues of chicken heart alive and well--not for just a few days, but for about twenty-eight years. That's almost twice the life of an ordinary hen.

These long-lived heart tissues were stored in a liquid which duplicated the heart's saline and mineral balance of sodium, potassium, calcium, glucose and several other nutrients supplying sufficient food for the tissue's growth. He changed the solution every day or so.

How did Dr. Carrel know these cardiac tissues were really alive? For one thing, they didn't decay. For another, they grew. (Had the heart tissue not been surgically separated from the animal's pituitary, which controls growth, the tissue would not have grown.)

In fact, these tissues expired only when Dr. Carrel stopped taking care of them--that is, when he stopped changing the solution at the necessary intervals.

He found no kind of "genetic clock" in such heart tissues forcing them to get old. With consistent care and correct feeding, reported this Nobel Prize-winner, these tissues were essentially immortal.

AGE DETERMINED BY BLOOD?

Further, said Dr. Carrel, the apparent "age of an

animal can be ascertained approximately by the growth index of its serum."

He meant blood serum, which is to say: The more efficiently--or quickly--serum in vitro (in a test tube) can grow new cells, the younger must be the donor of the serum; and the slower the serum, the older the donor.

What makes for the difference in these cellular speeds?

Too many of the wrong things fed into the serum slow down cell replication, Dr. Carrel said. Likewise, more of the right things (just so that "crowding" doesn't thicken the blood), the faster and more youthful the cellular replication.

This is a measure, then, of how quickly and efficiently and perfectly an organism (such as you or I) repairs itself.

It comes down to what kind of liquid or serum one has chosen in which to float his heart; what kind of "liquid" one has created for nurturing his heart, beat after beat, down the years.

We are talking, obviously, about the bloodstream. But we are trying to see it "in vitro"--in you, the human test-tube or petri dish.

Your bloodstream is your "solution." It is your creation. The serum therein metes out whatever repairs, replenishment of cells, you have provided; and therein lies much of the mystery of apparent age. Indeed, every man's and woman's body is his or her own private experimental laboratory; and the quality of their "solution" determines youthfulness or decrepitude.

"Longevity is only desirable if it increases the

duration of youth, and not that of old age. The length-
ening of the senescent period would be a calamity." --
Alexis Carrel, Man the Unknown (1935)

The only practical way, of course, to influence, to
change, or to create a perfect solution for your bodily
"petri dish" is through your liquids and diet. And we call
it food, whether or not it nurtures and feeds us properly.

According to Dr. Carrel, the worst offender
against cell replication in the test tube is lipoidal mat-
ter--that is, lipids. Fat.

WHY DIET IS CRITICAL

In other words, the truth about fat in blood serum
versus youth was well established in the year 1911,
when Dr. Carrel first made these observations. That
was eighty-five years ago! So it's hardly news.

At this point in time, remember, vitamins had not
been discovered. So unusable fat, thickening and
spoiling the bloodstream, was known about even
before we even knew about vitamins.

Can it be so large a step, then, to our seeing that
the main thing we do to the heart within us, the primary act which hurts the heart and shortens its life, is eating wrong foods? Like blindly putting the wrong fuel in
our gas tank?

Also harmful, in more rare cases, is eating too
much of the right food--flooding the engine.

FREE RADICALS AND HEART DISEASE

If a molecule has an electron that does not have a "partner," it becomes unstable and reactive--a free radical. To stabilize itself, it will steal an electron from a stable molecule.

One the stable molecule loses an electron, it, too, becomes a free radical. The second free radical steals an electron from a third molecule and so on--a destructive cycle has begun.

Each time a molecule loses an electron, it is damaged and will damage another molecule.

* How this affects you?

Our immune systems produce free radicals to destroy bacteria and viruses. When the body is invaded by harmful microorganisms, great numbers of free radicals are produced to try to overcome the infection. However, controlling the excessive flood of free radicals is vital to protect healthy tissues from damage.

So free radicals are vital for health. So they are not all bad. Only excessive and uncontrolled amounts of free radicals are damaging. But there is some speculation that excessive free radicals may start atherosclerosis by damaging blood vessel cells and lipoproteins. Lipids are especially susceptible to free radical attack, because electrons are less stable in lipids than in other types of molecules.

Lipoproteins, for the same reason, are very susceptible to free-radical damage. Responding to the damage, immune cells such as macrophages and platelets are sent to envelop the affected cells--which can result in plaque, a massive lump of cells. Damaged lipoproteins are also deposited in the plaque, along with the cholesterol they were carrying, which increases the plaque's size and stickiness. This again may block blood flow, leading to heart attacks, strokes and high blood pressure.

According to this theory, cholesterol itself is not the cause of the heart's problems, but an innocent bystander of free-radical damage. The distinction is between normal cholesterol and "oxidized" cholesterol, which has been damaged by free radicals.

Oxidized cholesterol is concentrated in plaques, and an elevated blood level shows that the body is losing the battle against free radicals.

Normal cholesterol, as has been noted, is a vital substance needed to maintain health. Only when free radicals damage or oxidize cholesterol does its presence increase heart-disease risk. So limiting dietary intake of cholesterol does not necessarily reduce that risk. More important is the effort to reduce the presence of excessive free radicals.

The free radical damage may actually lead to starvation of heart tissue, leading to severe pain (angina pectoris) and eventually heart attack itself.

ANTIOXIDANTS, FREE RADICALS & HEART DISEASE

A study of European middle-aged men by the World Health Organization found low blood levels of the antioxidant vitamin E to be a primary risk factor for death from heart disease--more important even than high blood pressure and high cholesterol levels.

Another study focused on the relationship between risk of angina pectoris and blood levels of the antioxidants vitamins A, C, E and carotene. Low levels of C, E and carotene were found to be significant factors in increased risk of angina, or heart pain. This was especially true for low levels of E.

The conclusion is that high-risk populations, and perhaps everybody, would benefit from diets rich in all antioxidants, but especially of vitamin E.

ANTIOXIDANTS AS ANTI-PLATELETS

In chapter two we discussed some of the dangers and side effects of antiplatelet drugs (see "Problems With Antiplatelets"). But antioxidant supplements can perform an antiplatelet role, without any of those negative effects.

To recap, platelets are blood cells responsible for clotting. If we didn't have them, a simple cut could cause massive bleeding. On the negative side, when platelets become too sticky or clot abnormally inside blood vessels, they can obstruct blood flow, starving body tissues of oxygen and food. If the tissues are in the brain, a stroke may result; in the heart, heart disease or even heart attack are possible consequences.

Clinical tests have found that antioxidant supplementation reduces platelet stickiness. In one controlled study (published in the American Journal of Clinical Nutrition, 1991), 78 men were given either a placebo or an antioxidant supplement (45,000 IU beta carotene, 600 mg vitamin C, 300 IU vitamin E and 75 mcg selenium) for five months. (Additional note on selenium: In one of many Dutch studies at Erasmus University Medical School, low levels of the mineral selenium were found in all cases of patients with atherosclerosis.)

Those receiving the placebo did not experience any lessening of platelet stickiness, but the antioxidant group had significant reduction in stickiness.

* More on Antioxidants and Plaque

A relatively new insight is that a high level of LDL cholesterol in and of itself may not lead to clogged arteries. It could be that before LDL can adhere to the flattened cells (called endothelial cells) that line your arteries, it has to be damaged by free radicals.

LDL cholesterol is packaged in fatty compartments called lipoproteins, which are prime targets for free-radical damage. When the lipoproteins become damaged, immune cells swarm to envelop them and cart them away. The result is a population of sticky globs of cholesterol that can cling to the linings of your arteries, forming swollen yellow mounds known as plaque. If other damaged lipoproteins add their cholesterol to the plaque, it can choke off the artery. (The surgical procedure called balloon angioplasty is designed to remove the plaque with an inflatable tool.)

Antioxidants reduce the oxidation of LDL cholesterol and prevent it from adhering to artery walls. In a recent study, a group of monkeys was fed a high-fat diet, and another group the same diet enriched with a potent antioxidant (probucol). The monkeys with the added antioxidant protection had much healthier arteries.

A study published in The Journal of the American Medical Association in 1995 showed that men who took at least 100 IU of vitamin E every day had less damage to their arteries than those who consumed smaller amounts of the antioxidant vitamin.

NON-PHARMACOLOGICAL PRINCIPLES

OF HEART HEALTH

There are nutrients, enzymes, anti-oxidants and other co-factors which, along with oxygen and "motion" that you yourself can put into your bloodstream, can and do restore youthfulness and health. These can and do act as a change of "saline solution" for your heart tissues.

We arrive then, at four basic ideas:

1. Retain your entire bloodstream. Don't let it start shrinking and closing down on you. Or narrowing, which is about the same thing.

2. Keep that bloodstream freshly supplied, every day.

3. Supply a proper balance of salts and minerals known to be natural and essential to heart chemistry (the heart's natural "bath"). And:

4: Include additional nutrients which will feed heart and all other tissues needing to be rebuilt--and rebuilt rapidly for youth, not slowly for decrepitude.

YOUR INCREDIBLE BLOODSTREAM

Before launching into the quick, easy things which you can do for your heart, we need to appreciate what an incredible system it is.

Your heart, when we speak of it, includes your entire circulatory system. And the full length of your bloodstream, your arteries and veins, your millions of capillaries, is approximately sixty-thousand miles--long enough to around the earth not once, but two and a half times!

And your blood, traveling this incredible journey,

doesn't require anything like the time it took Magellan to circumnavigate the world, which was years. Your blood travels along this unimaginable distance with every beat of your heart as if it were nothing at all.

The reason for seeing its vastness is so that you can appreciate fully the next incredible fact:

You could lose a hundred miles of bloodstream and scarcely know it. To have 59,900 miles of blood flow would seem to be about the same as 60,000. Then, mightn't you lose another 400 miles just as unconsciously? You'd still have 59,500 miles of bloodstream to keep you going, wouldn't you?

But these are not small losses.

And once you've lost them, can you get them back?

To grasp the vastness of these changes, picture the planet earth. Make the comparison:

Five-hundred miles of bloodstream equals the stretch of miles between the southernmost tip of California and the state capital, Sacramento, in the north. It equals the width of England--from Pembroke County to Essex. It equals the flight from London to Paris--and back.

Isn't it obvious that since you are born with this vast, incredible system, you must, for maximum health, use any and all means to get the blood flowing freely through all those miles, starving no tissues, losing no ground?

If you lose a hundred miles of capillaries due to agglutination, poor circulation, "couch potatoing," injury or your morning doughnut-and-coffee, something in you is not being fed. Something is being starved. Some continent of tissue, or island of crucial flesh which you'll need later (and will wish you'd kept alive, humming with vitality), is being taken away from you; and this is how we lose possession of ourselves, our inner "territories," our health, youthfulness and joy of living.

The heart will do its job all right, if something we do to it doesn't interfere. In fact, considering the strength, vitality and structure of the heart, as we have pointed out, it is ready to outlive us, instead of being the villain which lets us all down!

YOUR OTHER CIRCULATION SYSTEM

Your "other" bloodstream is the lymphatic system, the "clear" blood, which moistens your tissues, cleans them and rebuilds them. But it is a bloodstream without blood pressure. So, you may wonder, what pumps it?

The fact is that your movement--and nothing else--pumps the clear blood of your lymphatic system. Every drop of it has come from the arterial-venous system.

Here's how it works:

Red blood (including venous blood) leaks through the thin walls of the capillary system into intersticial tissues. Once this fluid--the very fluid of your bloodstream, minus red cells--has left the blood vessels, it is beyond the reach of your heart, except as a distant, quivering, rumbling kind of earthquake. Heart action does not pump this new form which your blood has taken.

EXERCISE: THE 'HEART' OF THE LYM-

PHATIC SYSTEM

The lymphatic system appears to have no particular "heart," but for your own arms and legs and motion. You pump this phase of the life of your bloodstream.

If you don't move around, your ankles swell, even hands and arms swell and become lethargic. Patients anchored to their beds, incapable of moving, must regularly be turned. For lymph settles. Gravity pulls the fluid, which is heavy, downward through your tissues.

Your heart needs this fluid, but has lost it. Yet while the fluid has leaked out--exited the control of blood pressure--its destination is not the lowest part of your body, but the upper part.

How, then, water being far heavier than fatty tissue, can this serum and lymph be raised upward to the level of the heart so that it may rejoin the bloodstream, pick up its red cells and be whole blood once again?

Again: Your own movements do the pumping. If you do not move, nothing gets pumped.

Further, since the heart depends upon this addition to its pool and needs it at every beat of your heart, it is necessary, it is urgent, that this lymph and serum be returned to its source as soon as possible, as quickly and easily as possible.

Easily? Especially as regards the heart. For every move you make, every breath you breathe, helps in some way to pump this pressure-less fluid back to your heart, back into the regular bloodstream.

WHAT LYMPH DOES

Billions of cells throughout your body require this lymphatic fluid. It carries the nutrients of your blood and feeds all other tissues.

Without a lively flow of blood serum, moisturizing and nurturing every cell, your tissues simply do not get fed.

If your tissues are not fed in this way, they starve.

But being active already, your cells form the byproducts of metabolism--that is, waste. As each cell is built and rebuilt, it has dross, which is cast off. These are toxins, waste materials which your body for the most part cannot use. Some wastes will, elsewhere, in other tissues, become recycled. The liver may, if working fully, convert lactic acid, the "fatigue" chemical of your muscles, back into useful fuel, giving long-distance runners an incredible sensation of "second wind."

The kidneys will remove iron for reuse, salvage some calcium or potassium, according to need; as also, the volume of water in the body is adjusted, its acid-alkaline balance moderated for health, and many other chemicals and toxins, indeed all the substances flowing through the arteries of the body must pass through the kidneys for approval or censure. These include certainly nutrients, minerals, proteins, acids, red cells, glucose and more.

But the more dangerous living bodies, as bacteria and virus (if indeed virus is alive), dangerous chemicals and every sort of infectious matter are fought and if possible destroyed by the lymphatic system (though also by the liver and spleen).

The greater part of the human body is not penetrated by blood vessels. And thus, it is this greater mass of tissue that must be cleaned, germ-proofed, chemically balanced and fed by serum.

Even more important, fats are mostly carried by the lymph, and made safe chemically (if not mechanically) for entering the heart at the vena cava, the two large veins conveying blood to the right atrium.

Fats, in the form of digested oils, are then, by this mechanism, dumped directly into the blood and, in fact, into the heart. So they must be made safe--and this toil, again of cleaning things up, falls upon the lymphatic system, your "second bloodstream," heroic, unsung and crucial to life and the quality of your health.

HOW THE LYMPHATIC SYSTEM AFFECTS HEART HEALTH

It is this serum about which Dr. Alexis Carrel was speaking when he wrote that age was virtually defined by the vitality of this serum to do its feeding and make its repairs.

It is this same fluid, the serum, which Dr. Carrel discovered must be kept fresh, clean and almost constantly changing to keep heart tissue virtually immortal. But allow this serum to grow foul in any way, and death quickly follows.

We are talking about the health of the heart.

The heart, to begin with, is already healthy. It does not poison itself, but may become poisoned. And the poisoning begins with serum, which is, in turn, "created" from wrong materials, and which does not circulate by sufficient movement--activity by the person--to be, in fact "fresh."

All that is needed to begin the slow poisoning and premature death of heart tissue is to slow down the change of this serum. Even nutritionally strong serum, if unchanged, allows heart tissue to die.

So exercise not only doesn't cause stress to the heart, it recreates and rests it, refreshes and feeds it.

Our bodies are that missing lymphatic heart, and its ventricals are our arms and legs. With deep and long respiration pulling poisons from the lungs, with carefree, repetitive physical activity--running, jumping, dancing, swimming--this crucial and vital serum of your second bloodstream is pumped rapidly through the intersticial tissues where either life or death is made.

HOW EXERCISE 'RESTS' THE HEART

The fact is that one cannot merely "have a healthy heart." The healthy heart is a heart that is cared for by an active person who grasps the strange fact that activity of the limbs both rests and protects the heart.

Inactivity, no matter how carefully rationalized, brings death to the heart. This organ was made to function as we see it in living creatures. The heart was not made to stop. The heart scarcely knows how to stop and is brought to a stop only by force.

Yet, the heart has its methods for rest. It rests between beats, it slows down at night and, when all minerals are present, takes its ease with soft, easy beats.

Yet "rest" of mere inactivity during waking hours is not what strengthens and rebuilds the heart.

* There are three basic kinds of rest known to the heart, and which should be supplied by anyone who seeks long and comfortable years. The "rests" of the heart are these:

1. The heart's own relaxation between beats;

2. Slowness and softness during wholesome, nourished sleep; and--

3. Rhythmic, deliberate activity which restores the "other" bloodstream--fresh serum--to its source, directly into the heart.

MORE TIPS TO HELP YOUR LYMPHATIC SYSTEM

The only time you are likely be aware of your lymph system is when you had a sore throat or other infection, and felt enlarged lymph nodes in your neck or armpit or groin. These little pea-shaped organs are part of a network of delicate vessels throughout your body that transport the lymphatic fluid.

Lymph, as we've outlined, is a clear or milky fluid that originates in the blood capillaries, leaking out into the spaces between the cells. Inside the cells, fluids serve to transport nourishment and carry away wastes.

Each cell is surrounded by a permeable membrane that allows materials to pass through to the outside. The fluid that bathes the outside of the cells is the lymph. Waste materials pass out of the cells, and out of the bloodstream through the capillary walls, and are eventually picked up by the lymph vessels. After traveling a short distance, these lymph vessels enter lymph nodes.

The major lymph nodes are concentrated in the groin, armpits, neck, chest, and abdomen. Within specialized compartments in the lymph nodes are found different white cells, such as lymphocytes and macrophages, which have important functions in the immune system, protecting your body from infection and foreign materials.

The lymphocytes circulate throughout the lymph system and attack invading organisms. When your body is fighting an infection, the lymph nodes become swollen near the site of the infection, as the bacteria are carried to the nodes, where they are engulfed and gobbled up by the macrophages. The lymph nodes also contain webbed areas that filter the lymph, removing foreign materials. After the lymph has been filtered, it leaves the lymph node, carrying the freshly cleaned lymph out the other side.

The lymph vessels have valves, which allow the fluid to flow in only one direction, toward the heart. The lymph flow rejoins the bloodstream at the base of the neck, where the largest lymphatic collecting vessel, the thoracic duct, empties its lymph into the internal jugular vein to mix with the blood.

Normal lymph is a watery fluid, and it must remain at the proper consistency in order to move readily through its vessels. Certain kinds of debris and toxic materials cause the lymph to become thick or mucoidlike in consistency.

* Keeping Lymph Clear

As we discussed, exercise is another very important factor in keeping your lymph clear. While your blood is moved through the body by the pumping action of your heart, the lymph system depends on the contraction of the muscles surrounding the vessels to keep it moving along. Muscular contractions increase pressure within the system, causing the valves to close; when pressure decreases, the valves open and the lymph flows. When the body is not moving, the lymph in the arms, legs, and head does not move measurably. With activity, drainage of the lymph system increases tenfold.

Some kinds of exercise are better than others for moving the lymph through the system. All vigorous exercise, such as brisk walking with strongly swinging arms, is beneficial in moving the lymph.

* Foot Soaks and Your Lymph

Soaking your feet helps to open the pores and draw the toxins out of the lymph system through the skin. The Romans knew the value of bathing the feet in the waters of their healing springs, and at the great French spas, footbaths were the prescribed treatment for arthritis. The effects of footbaths are aided by specific minerals or herbs added to the water, and by the temperature of the water itself.

* Lymphatic Massage

After your foot soak, an excellent way to continue lymphatic stimulation is through massage. Remember that the lymph flows toward the heart-up from the feet and down from the head.

Lower-Body Lymphatic Massage

Massage one leg at a time. Using one or two hands, begin by massaging at the base of each toe and between the toes. Massage gently in a circular motion; imagine yourself loosening the toxins and debris from all the tiny lymph vessels between your toes.

After you have gently massaged the base of

each toe, stroke upward with both hands, drawing the lymph up and toward the ankles with a gentle, feathery, upward stroking motion. Move up to the ankle; gently massage in a circular motion all around the ankle, and then lightly stoke upward, drawing the lymph up the calf until you get to the knee.

Massage with both hands all around the knee, over the lymph nodes behind the knee, and around the kneecap, in circular motions. Use light pressure; this is the best way to stimulate the lymph. Remember that the lymph vessels are close to the surface of the skin. Draw the lymph up along the thighs, using the fingertips or the palms of the hands. At the back of the thigh, massage gently at the base of the buttock, in a gentle circular motion; this is one of the areas where the toxic waste of cellulite tends to accumulate.

Stroke upward, along the thigh, and bring it all around and back into the groin. After you have completed one leg, work on the other leg.

In the groin area, work on both sides at once. Stroke upward and diagonally across the groin area with the flat of the hand on each side, moving the hands toward each other so they come together over the abdomen. Repeat this upward stroking all along the groin area; there are many lymph nodes in this area.

As you stroke gently upward and into the abdominal area, picture all the debris and waste being moved along, to be absorbed and eliminated through your colon.

When you do a lymphatic massage, you may notice that some areas react painfully to pressure. Most women, for example, if they press hard between their breasts, will feel a very sensitive spot. This is one of the areas where lymph congestion can produce tenderness. If a woman finds such a sensitive spot, she should not be afraid to touch it; continue to gently massage it with a light, circular motion, and then, with a feathery touch, move it onward-up from the legs, down from the head.

You will notice that there is less and less lymphatic congestion and that you have fewer sensitive spots. Spend about ten minutes on the lymphatic massage. Proper lymphatic functioning produces clear, glowing skin; and, because it is a vital part of your immune system, it helps to promote your resistance to disease.

* Upper-Body Lymph Massage

This gentle upper-body self-massage helps to flush congested lymph out of the extremities and toward the heart, where it joins the main lymph drainage of the body.

Begin your massage at the neck, under the chin, in the areas where you may have sometimes noticed swollen lymph glands. Massage with the fingertips from ear to ear in a gentle circular motion, then gently stroke from the ears under the chin toward the center.

Now, with your fingertips, gently stroke downward, from under the chin down the neck. Use these gentle downward stroking movements all around the neck, moving the lymph from beneath the chin and the base of the skull down into the top of your chest.

Next, using your left hand, work on the right arm, beginning at the wrist. Use your fingers to repeatedly smooth and stroke the inside of the arm, from the wrist up to the inner elbow. When you reach the inside of the elbow, gently massage with a circular motion, then continue with a light, feathery, stroking movement up the inside of the arm to the underarm.

In the armpit area, gently squeeze with thumb and fingers, releasing the lymph and moving it up and out of the arm. This is another area where many lymph nodes are located, and where you may have noticed swelling when you have been sick.

Women should stroke from the armpit up over the top of the right breast, using light, feathery strokes to bring the lymph out of the armpit and around toward the center of the chest. Guide the lymph from the right shoulder, the right arm area, and the neck, all down toward the middle of the chest.

Then use the right hand and repeat this process, bringing the lymph up the left arm and into the armpit. Concentrate a little longer on the left side, to work the lymph out of the armpit and along the extensive lymph drainage around the heart. Draw it all in toward the center of the chest, into the area between the breasts.

Next, women should rub in a gentle circular motion between the breasts. It is quite possible to feel some tenderness in this area; this simply means that there is some lymph congestion here. Do not be alarmed; just continue to gently massage, and over time the congestion will begin to be relieved. Now, massage beneath the breasts, about an inch or so below each breast, stroking gently around the bottom of the breasts toward the middle, bringing it all down into the abdomen. Stroke gently downward all the way across your chest beneath your breasts, moving the lymph into the abdomen, where the waste will be eliminated by the colon.

HOW TO EXERCISE YOUR HEART

See the next chapter!

Notes:

_____

_____

_____

_____

_____

_____

_____

_____

_____

V. HEARTY EXERCISE

THE MOST IMPORTANT THING YOU CAN DO FOR YOUR HEART

This chapter connects with the introduction-- remember, those "Nine Easy Steps to Heart Health"? The first and most important of these, you may recall, was exercise, the one you should do if you could do only one.

"A journey of a thousand miles begins with...

a little sweat." -- variation of Chinese proverb

SOME BENEFITS OF EXERCISE

Regular physical exercise can and should play a key role in your effort to reduce the risk of heart disease. Here are some of the benefits of such a program:

1. Improved cholesterol levels.

Bad LDL cholesterol is brought down with ongoing exercise. HDL levels go up. Better yet, the more one exercises and the more strenuous that exercise becomes, the greater the gain in HDL. And, thanks to the weight loss that typically accompanies a long-term exercise program, LDL and total cholesterol both come down. (See "HOW MUCH EXERCISE TO RAISE HDL?" below.)

2. Weight loss.

Not only does this take place by burning off

stored fat, but by using up calories that might otherwise be stored as fat. Also, the metabolism continues to be elevated for hours after exercise, so you'll be able to consume more food without gaining weight.

3. Lower blood pressure.

Like the cholesterol-lowering effect, this benefit, too, is measurable only over a period of time. But scientific data substantiate the claim that regular exercise can control mild to moderate hypertension without the need for drugs. More amazing, even patients with severely elevated blood pressure may lessen their medication requirement through habitual exercise.

4. Improved heart and lung fitness.

Heart: The heart normally pumps about six quarts of blood a minute. But during vigorous exercise, blood volume to and from the heart rises to about 25 quarts per minute. The extra labor strengthens the heart muscle.

And those who exercise on a regular basis are protecting themselves against the tendency of the blood platelets to form clots. Some scientists believe that vigorous exercise can promote the formation of new arterial pathways--tiny collateral arteries that provide a kind of natural bypass around clogged arteries.

Indeed, evidence is accumulating that regular exercise may not only help you prevent heart attacks, but help you recover faster if you do suffer a heart attack.

Lungs: The increased lung fitness takes place by what is often called the training effect--increasing the capacity to utilize oxygen in several ways.

Without oxygen, of course, cells die and organs cease to work. Four minutes without oxygen causes irreversible brain damage. A heart attack is simply what happens when heart tissue is denied oxygen.

By strengthening the muscles of respiration (the chest and abdominal muscles that expand the rib cage), the flow of air in and out of the lungs is facilitated--and the system receives more life-giving oxygen.

The outflow of air is often overlooked, by the way, but it, too, is critically important. When the rib cage returns to normal size, exhalation of air depends upon the ability of the lungs to contract by themselves and push out the remaining air. Often, with age and infirmity, this elasticity is lost. (And coughing, as smokers experience, will also aggravate this weakness.) The depleted air that is not expelled from the lungs dilutes the fresh air inhaled and can lead to chronic oxygen deprivation or starvation.

5. Control of diabetes.

Exercise accomplishes this by helping to stabilize blood sugar levels. Regular physical activity, with an insulin-like effect, can nearly eliminate the symptoms and health risks of type II, non-insulin-dependent diabetes.

6. Improved psychological health.

A person who keeps physically fit usually experiences a sense of well-being that can spread to other areas of life--and help performance under stressful conditions. And those who learn to make exercise a habit often increase self-esteem by setting and attaining their exercise goals.

There is also a "feel-good" effect to aerobic exercise, traceable to certain body chemicals known as endorphins. These blunt pain and induce a mild euphoria. Endorphins are produced in the spinal cord and the brain, and are the reason, some theorize, that exercise seems to lessen anxiety and stress.

7. Increased flexibility.

This is an often overlooked benefit to exercise, helping to protect the muscles against pulls and tears.

8. Improved sleep.

Steady exercise stimulates the release of the chemical serotonin, one of the neurotransmitters, which helps to promote sleep. Pharmaceutical companies, in fact, have been attempting to incorporate serotonin in their tranquilizing medications. By exercising, you'll be getting your serotonin naturally.

9. Increased longevity.

This outlandish-sounding claim turns out to be pretty well substantiated. More than one recent study has correlated physical fitness programs with longer life-spans. One report published in the Journal of the American Medical Association in 1995 showed that the more strenuous the activity, the greater the gain in longevity.

BONUS BENEFIT OF EXERCISE

Another little-known but dramatic benefit of the right type of exercise is an improvement to the immune system. How does this occur? Exercise causes the release of growth hormone from the brain's pituitary gland. Growth hormone helps stimulate the immune system, while building muscles and burning fats.

Note: This growth hormone release diminishes

dramatically with age.

HOW MUCH EXERCISE TO RAISE HDL?

Several studies have indicated that regular exercise can raise the level of the "good cholesterol," HDL. But how much exercise is enough?

A recent Georgetown University study suggests that a moderate amount of jogging or brisk walking should be beneficial for middle-aged and older people. Volunteers were nearly 3,000 healthy, nonsmoking men between the ages of 30 and 64 who passed a treadmill test and were of normal weight and average fitness for their age. The men filled out a health questionnaire, underwent a physical examination that included measurement of cholesterol levels, then were divided into six groups on the basis of the number of miles they ran weekly (none, 3-6, 7-10, 11-14, 15-20, or more than 20 miles per week).

The results revealed a definite relationship between the amount of exercise and HDL level: the greater the amount of exercise, the higher the HDL. HDL-cholesterol levels were higher (by about 0.3 mg/dl) for every mile run. Most increases occurred in men who ran from 7 to 14 miles weekly, at rates of about 10-11 minutes per mile, for a weekly total of about 1 1/2 to 2 hours.

Such exercise levels are easily matched by a moderate jog or brisk walk of about 30 minutes three to five times a week. The group who jogged between 11 and 14 miles per week had an HDL cholesterol level 11% higher and an LDL cholesterol 8% lower than the nonexercising group.

Long-term effects:

Other studies have suggested that significant increases in HDL cholesterol can occur from a month to a year after people begin regular exercise.

WHAT HAPPENS WHEN YOU EXERCISE?

During sedentary periods, you take about 10 to 14 breaths a minute, receiving about 9 to 12 pints of air. During vigorous, sustained exercise, however, you inhale 20 or more times a minute, taking in around 20 gallons a minute.

The equation is simple: the amount of air you breathe depends upon your body's oxygen demands. (The signal for more oxygen is sent by your muscles to the brain, which orders the heart to pump harder and the blood pressure to rise.

HOW DO YOU 'FLEX' THE HEART MUSCLE?

Exercising the biceps muscle is easy. You work directly on it, doing dumbbell or barbell curls. But you can't do the same with the cardiac muscle--flexing and contracting directly. Since we don't exercise conscious control over this muscle, we have to work it indirectly.

The trick is working other muscle groups for a sustained period of time. This automatically works the heart harder to supply those muscles with blood. And the increased carbon dioxide in the blood--from burning fuel--forces the lungs to work harder. And increasing pumping of the heart requires a increased resiliency in the entire vascular system--creating a greater variety of routes for the blood to flow from the heart to the muscle and back again.

But for the essential "training effect" to occur, there has to be a certain duration of effort.

WHY MANY SPORTS HAVE LITTLE OR NO TRAINING EFFECT

Playing football or baseball may be fun and leave you sweaty and exhausted, yet offer little training effect. That's because it's too intermittent--there's too much stopping and starting and standing around between plays.

Sprinting a hundred yards, for instance, requires an effort both too great and too brief to be of lasting value.

Those who excel in these sports, of course, need to be well conditioned. But more and more they must get their training effects elsewhere--via weight resistance programs or aerobic exercise.

The best sports for cardiovascular training are those that require constant activity with a minimum of pauses. Examples: soccer, basketball, tennis, handball. The reasons why one type of activity is more conducive to heart health than another have to do with oxygen utilization--their "aerobic" factor.

AEROBIC VS. NONAEROBIC EXERCISE

There are two basic types of exercise: aerobic and anaerobic. "Aerobic" is derived from a Greek word meaning "air." Dr. Kenneth Cooper, who devised the first aerobic programs for the U.S. Air Force, defined it as any variety of exercise that stimulates heart and lung activity for a sufficient time to produce beneficial changes in the body.

Aerobic exercise means exercise "with oxygen."

An aerobic exercise ("without air") is designed to strengthen individual muscles. By making exertions that require more oxygen than breathing can supply, muscles go into "oxygen debt," drawing on their own stored resources. This builds muscle mass, but does not improve cardiovascular function.

If you're more concerned with burning excess body fat for energy, and not with building strength or lean body mass, then aerobic exercise is what you want.

PUMPING IRON AND HDL?

Despite what we've just said, there is interesting evidence that one nonaerobic activity, weight training, may contribute to a lowering of cholesterol.

Forty-six women were tested by researchers at the Department of Veteran Affairs Medical Center and the University of Arizona, both in Tucson. These women enrolled in a weight-training program, exercising for an hour three times a week. A second group of women continued with their normal exercise programs, thereby acting as a control group.

Five months later, the women pumping iron had their total cholesterol drop from 184 to 171 milligrams/deciliter. Even better, their "bad" LDL cholesterol dropped 12 percent, from 116 to 102 milligrams/deciliter, without significantly affecting their HDL levels.

Pass the dumbbell please.

EXERCISE-OF-THE-MONTH CLUB

Because of their aerobic benefits, certain forms of exercise--many of them noncompetitive--are much better than competitive sports for heart health. Dr. Cooper headed his aerobic list with running, swimming, cycling, jogging, but there are many others, of course, including aerobic dance, stair-climbing, step classes, cross-country skiing and rowing.

(See chart below, "Aerobic Activities Rated," with estimated hourly rate of calories "burned.")

Which aerobic exercise is best for you? Because of individual factors, there can be no ultimate answer. Every month, it seems, brings new studies by exercise physiologists and cardiologists, pointing now to walking or jogging, now to aerobic calisthenics or stationary exercise equipment.

Obviously, it's important for you to select an activity that you can accommodate realistically into your lifestyle, one that you will enjoy--and, more particularly, enjoy on a continuing basis. If you use a rowing machine, let's say, for three times a week for a half-hour at a time, by the end of a year you'll have rowed about 78 hours--about two weeks of a typical work schedule. So you'd better pick something you like!

Which is one recommendation for the most basic of all aerobic activities--one easy, safe and enjoyable--namely walking.

WALKING FIT

One frequent prescription, as has been noted, is to exercise for longer periods of time, but at less than a maximum heart rate. The best exercise for this is walking.

Walking at an average clip, as you'll see on the "calorie burn" chart, uses slightly more than 300 calories per hour. Even walking at a very slow pace will burn 80 calories per hour. Walking at an average speed six hours per week--less than an hour per day--will burn all the calories you need to get the beneficial training effect.

It will also help you lose or moderate your weight. Visit any country where the citizenry is forced to walk at least an hour a day, and you'll see very few "plumpy dumplings."

Another way to look at it: walking a mile burns only about 1.5 percent fewer calories than jogging the same distance.

Other advantages to walking: the risk of injury is much less than with walking or even slow jogging. Moreover, walking can be done anywhere at any time and stimulates a natural rhythm which can clear the mind of stress and help you relax. If you're not experiencing this, look around and smell the roses or at least enjoy the scenery.

* Getting started:

You might consider a regular walking program that starts as a 15-minute walk three times a week. The first 5 minutes of the walk should be taken at a moderate pace. This warm-up should be followed by brisk walking for 5 minutes so that the heart reaches its "target zone."

(**Note:** You can increase the aerobic benefits of your workout by swinging your arms vigorously--or by doing so with light arm or hand weights; see section on "Power-Walking" below.)

During a final 5-minute period, the pace should become slower again. In the following weeks and months, 2 minutes a day can be added to the brisk-walking segment, so that by the 12th week brisk walking lasts for 30 minutes and by the 28th it lasts for one hour.

You can also step up this program is by walking five times per week, instead of three. Or intensify the workout by "heading for the hills." You'll burn more calories and your heart will work harder as you tackle an incline. In fact, even walking downhill will force your heart to work harder than on a level surface.

Caution: Before setting off on this trek toward heart health, make sure you have good footwear. You don't have to spend big bucks on the trendiest walking shoes. You do need a rigid arch with cushioning at the heel and ball of the foot. (More on this in the next section.)

POWER-WALKING

The famous bodybuilder Steve Reeves wrote a book on "PowerWalking" (Bobbs-Merrill). Check it out of the library and read it. Reeves recommends you stretch your legs. Swing your arms. Almost run. Be sure that no part of your body is tense, so all parts are equally exercised.

Protect your heels, arches, leg muscles and all joints, from your ankles to your neck, by "double-socking." First, rub a reasonably thick lotion, oil or lanolin on your feet. Put on two pair of gym socks, then your walking/jogging shoes.

Dress warmly enough that a sudden breeze won't give your perspiring body a chill. Exercise sufficiently to work up a wholesome sweat. (Walking around in your house won't do this. Besides, you need to get out.)

When possible, jog or power-walk on grass or ground rather than on concrete. Black-top is better than cement (unless the sun's hot, and the tarmac is melty, sticking to your shoes and sending up petroleum vapors).

Of course, even though you've got the right of way, yield to fast-moving cars and trucks by walking in circles till you've got the green light. Yes, some car-bound folks will think you're bonkers, spinning with one wing dropped. Who cares? Laugh and wave, but keep moving.

PROTECT YOURSELF ON THE GO

Wear dark glasses to prevent ultraviolet damage to your eyes (and, perhaps if you're really overweight, so your skinny neighbors won't know who you are).

On hot days, wear a sweatband. If the sun is overhead, you might consider protecting both hair and the top of your head from serious sun damage. Under your cap, inside the crown, you can attach a piece of red cloth and one of green cloth. Explorers in the tropic regions discovered that even their solar pith helmets didn't protect them from sunstroke unless they wore these red-and green-colored cloths.

These details may seem picky; but you want the maximum benefit and the least penalty. Take precautions ahead of time, then be carefree while out walking.

A walking companion offers another dimension. But don't get into the habit of calling off the outing when someone else defaults.

A running track provides you with soil (or rubberized surface) instead of cement and a means of measuring the length of your walk. The rules of the road apply here--slow joggers keep right.

On the road, try to avoid high vehicular traffic because of exhaust fumes, which, unfortunately, are absorbed by the lungs 17 times more readily than is clear air. When hitting a cloud of bad air or dust, hold your breath for a few paces--but not too long, of course. You don't want to black-out.

In very warm dry climates, many sports-minded folk tuck a lightweight plastic bottle of water fortified with electrolytes (trace minerals) or some kind of sports drink inside their belt or in a pocket. You can sip this restoring drink along the way if you feel dehydrated.

AVOIDING DEHYDRATION AND ELECTROLYTE DEPLETION

It's not necessary to take salt, even if you sweat a lot, but replacing trace minerals is a must. You can buy highly concentrated trace minerals in your health-food store; add them to your drink. You should know, however, that a thoroughly salt-free diet can lead to exhaustion.

As mentioned elsewhere, salt nurtures the adrenal glands, and a shortage can cause people to pass out. This has happened. Even though our foods generally supply sufficient sodium, pedestrians have strangely passed out right on the pavement. Emergency care and examination have disclosed that these unfortunate victims thought they were doing right to avoid all salt.

A general principle: Don't avoid anything of proved, long-term value. Instead, learn the moderate and best amounts for you.

After all these precautions and hints, don't let all these preliminary considerations turn you off. You need to move, to move rhythmically, to go fast and work up a steaming sweat. Every step you take helps to push your blood serum and lymph up through all your intersticial ti sues, and return these essential life-givers to your heart.

So remember: exercise feeds your heart the most wonderful food of all--serum (as immunizing, lymphatic fluid) rich in all nutrients, except oxygen. And your lungs provide that. So breath with gusto. Enjoy gasping a lot.

* Special note for especially lazy folks: Yes, without exercise your heart goes on beating. But a life of inactivity starves and stresses the heart.

PAIN IS NOT GAIN

There are all kinds of excuses for abandoning an exercise regimen. But one of the most common is because a person tries to do too much too soon and gets hurt. "No pain, no gain" may apply to some forms of athleticism, but not aerobic exercise. Effort is one thing; discomfort is another. Pain is a warning sign that your muscles are being strained. If an exercise hurts repeatedly, stop doing it--and don't start again until you can do it without of injury.

KEEP YOUR EXERCISE PROGRAM AFLOAT

Many people find that an "exercise companion" increases motivation and helps with follow-through. A little amicable competition and companionship can make the difference between activity and inertia. Others ensure that they will exercise by writing it into their calendar. General advice: If you can't talk comfortably during brisk physical activity, it's too vigorous. Reduce the intensity.

Warning: Anyone who experiences chest pain, feels faint or lightheaded or becomes extremely out of breath while exercising should stop the activity at once and contact a doctor as soon as possible. Other symptoms which should cause alarm: headache, dizziness, discomfort or numbness in the jaw, neck or arm.

5 WAYS TO AVOID SPORTS INJURIES

The American Heart Association gives the following tips to cut down exercise injuries:

1. Build up your level of activity gradually. Try not to set your goals too high--otherwise you will be tempted to push yourself too far too quickly. For activities such as jogging, walking briskly and jumping rope, limber up gently and slowly before and after exercising. For other activities, build up slowly to your target zone, and cool down slowly afterwards.

2. Listen to your body for early warning pains. Exercising too much can cause injuries to joints, feet, ankles and legs. Don't make the mistake of exercising beyond early warning pains in these areas or more serious injuries may result. Fortunately, minor muscle and joint injuries can be readily treated by rest and aspirin.

3. Be aware of possible signs of heart problems such as: Pain or pressure in the left or mid-chest area, left neck, shoulder or arm during or just after exercising. (Vigorous exercise may cause a side stitch while exercising--a pain below your bottom ribs - which is not the result of a heart problem.)

Sudden lightheartedness, cold sweat, pallor or fainting. Ignoring these signals and continuing to exercise may lead to serious heart problems. Should any of these signs occur, stop exercising and call your doctor.

4. For outdoor activities, take appropriate precautions under special weather conditions. On hot, humid days:

--Exercise during the cooler and/or less humid parts of the day such as early morning or early evening after the sun has gone down.

--Exercise less than normal for a week until you become adapted to the heat.

--Drink lots of fluids, particularly water--before, during and after exercising. Usually, you do not need extra salt because you get enough salt in your diet. (And a well-conditioned body is better able to conserve salt so that most of the sweat is water.)

But if you exercise very vigorously for an extended time in the heat (for example, running a marathon), it's a good idea to increase your salt intake a little.

--Watch out for signs of heat stroke--feeling dizzy, weak, light-headed, and/or excessively tired; sweating stops; or body temperature becomes dangerously high.

--Wear a minimum of light, loose-fitting clothing.

--Avoid rubberized or plastic suits, sweatshirts and sweat pants. Such clothing will not actually help you lose weight any faster by making you sweat more. The weight you lose in fluids by sweating will be quickly replaced as soon as you begin drinking fluids again. This type of clothing can also cause dangerously high temperatures, possibly resulting in heat stroke.

On cold days:

--Wear one layer less of clothing than you would wear if you were outside but not exercising. It's also better to wear several layers of clothing rather than one heavy layer. You can always remove a layer if you get too warm.

--Use old mittens, gloves, or cotton socks to protect your hands.

--Wear a hat, since up to 40 percent of your body's heat is lost through your neck and head.

On rainy, icy or snowy days:

--Be aware of reduced visibility (for yourself and

for drivers) and reduced traction on pathways.

5. Other handy tips are:

--If you've eaten a meal, avoid strenuous exercise for at least 2 hours. If you exercise vigorously first, wait about 20 minutes before eating.

--Use proper equipment such as goggles to protect your eyes for handball or racquetball, or good shoes with adequate cushioning in the soles for running or walking.

--Hard or uneven surfaces such as cement or rough fields are more likely to cause injuries. Soft, even surfaces such as a level grass field, a dirt path, or a track for running are better for your feet and joints.

--If you run or jog, land on your heels rather than the balls of your feet. This will minimize the strain on your feet and lower legs.

--Joggers or walkers should also watch for cars and wear light- colored clothes with a reflecting band during darkness so that drivers can see you. Remember, drivers don't see you as well as you see their cars. Face oncoming traffic and do not assume that drivers will notice you on the roadway.

--If you bicycle, you can help prevent injuries by always wearing a helmet and using lights and wheel-mounted reflectors at night. Also, ride in the direction of traffic and try to avoid busy streets.

--Check your shopping malls. Many malls are open early and late for people who do not wish to exercise alone in the dark. They also make it possible to be active in bad weather and to avoid summer heat, winter cold or allergy seasons.

START SLOW FOR SUCCESS

Not ready to start a daily walking regimen? Don't be discouraged. Remember, any activity is going to be a significant improvement over no activity.

The objective of any aerobic exercise regimen is to increase the amount of oxygen your body can take in and process in a given period of time. But conditioning cannot occur overnight, and people who have not exercised for a long time should take a gradual approach.

As a first step, they can build physical activity into their daily routine--by taking a regular walk each day or by using the stairs instead of the elevator. They can get off the bus one or two stops before their destination, park some distance from a store, trade coffee breaks for walk breaks, use a bike for errands or work in the yard or garden.

One medical study found that such moderate exercise--just 30 minutes a day of light activity like walking or gardening--is nearly as beneficial to one's health as higher levels of exercise, like aerobics or jogging. And moderate exercise is far safer than high-intensity aerobics, especially for those entrenched in sedentary ways or already diagnosed with heart disease.

**AEROBIC ACTIVITIES RATED
BURNING CALORIES**

ACTIVITY	CALORIES BURNED*

Bicycling 6 mph	240
Bicycling 12 mph	410
Cross-country skiing	700
Jogging 5 1/2 mph	740
Jogging 7 mph	920
Jumping rope	750
Running in place	650
Running 10 mph	1280
Swimming 25 yds/min	275
Swimming 50 yds/min	500
Tennis--singles	400
Walking 2 mph	240
Walking 3 mph	320
Walking 4 1/2 mph	440

* Average calories burned by a 150-pound person per hour. A lighter person burns fewer calories; a heavier person burns more.

WALK THE FAIRWAY FOR FITNESS

You can reap the benefits of exercise without embarking on some approved physical fitness regimen. One Purdue University study found that eighteen holes of golf (where the golfer walked and carried his or her own clubs) was equivalent to running six miles--or burning 660 calories more each hour than just sitting in front of a TV. Digging in a garden, meanwhile, came in at 540 calories per hour, pushing a lawnmower at 470.

BURNING CALORIES WHILE KNOCKING DOWN PINS

Bowling is not usually grouped among advanced cardiovascular activities. But it is certainly physical activity, as the 5 million league bowlers in the United States (and 116 million abroad) can attest. And emerging research indicates that it brings considerable health benefits. Among them:

1. Calorie-burning. A 125-pound person burns about 205 calories per hour bowling; a 150-pound person, 245; a 175-pound person, 285. That's about the same as slow dancing or playing golf without a cart.

But since bowling is usually done in a group, alternating activity and rests, a person usually must bowl three hours to get one full hour of actual activity. But there's less down time than in downhill skiing, for instance, where it can often take about five hours on the slope to equal one full hour of skiing.

2. Weight-lifting. In a typical three-game series, a bowler would swing a 12- to 16-pound ball 36 to 63 times, which would be the equivalent of lifting up to nearly half a ton, according to Mark Miller of Bowling Headquarters, a Milwaukee-based membership organization.

That may equate to some increase in muscle tone, but only in the arm you use for bowling.

3. Rest and relaxation. One of the key benefits of any exercise programs, along with cardiovascular and muscular conditioning, is better sleep afterward. And bowlers often experience such benefits.

4. Stress-reduction. There's something about knocking those pins silly--or even coming close--that gets rid of accumulated aggression, bowlers say.

5. Low injury risk. Sore thumbs are the most common complaint, followed by muscle pulls in the shoulders and back. To reduce risk, find a ball that fits well; stretch beforehand.

6. Improved eye-hand coordination. There is no guarantee of this, of course, but there's a great incentive to work on such coordination. If not, you're going to keep scoring poorly.

7. Improved social life. Bowling is rarely a solitary sport, and it's fun to do in a group.

EXERCISE IN YOUR TARGET HEART-RATE ZONE

A person's maximum heart rate is the fastest his or her heart can beat. Exercise above 75% of one's maximum heart rate may be too strenuous, but exercise below 50% is of little benefit to the heart and lungs. The best activity level is 50-75% of this maximum heart rate--a range called a person's target heart-rate zone.

Beginners in an exercise program should aim for the lower part (50-60%) of their target zone during the first few months. Over the next six months, they can gradually build up to 75%--and beyond, if they choose--although they can stay in good condition without exercising that hard. Some blood-pressure-lowering drugs also lower the maximum heart rate and thus the target-zone rate. People who are taking such medications should call their physician to find out whether to adjust their exercise program. Patients with pacemakers should ask their doctor if there are any restrictions on exercise.

To determine whether you are exercising at the appropriate level, take your pulse immediately after exercise. Place the tips of the first two fingers lightly over one of the blood vessels on the neck (carotid arteries), located to the left or right of Adam's apple, or on the inside of the wrist just below the base of the thumb. Then count the pulse for 15 seconds and multiply by 4. If the pulse falls within your target zone, then you are at the appropriate level of exercise. If it is below your target zone, then you should exercise a little harder next time; if it is above your target zone, you should exercise a little easier. Once you are exercising within your target zone, you should check your pulse at least once a week during the first three months and periodically after that to make sure you are exercising at the right intensity.

TARGET ZONES BY AGE

Age in Years	Avg. Maximum Heart Rate (100%)	Target Heart-Rate Zone (50-75%)	
	Beats per Minute	Beats per Minute	Beats per 15 Seconds

20	200	100-150	25-38
25	195	98-146	24-37
30	190	95-142	24-36
35	185	93-138	23-35
40	180	90-135	23-34
45	175	88-131	22-33
50	170	85-127	21-32
55	165	83-123	21-31
60	160	80-120	20-30
65	155	78-116	19-29
70	150	75-113	18-28

The maximum heart rate is approximately 220 minus age. The table figures are averages and are general guidelines. To find your target zone, look for the age category closest to your age and read the line across. For example, if you are 50, your target zone is 85-127 beats per minute or 21-32 beats for each 15-second period. If you are 63, the closest age on the chart is 65; the target zone is 78-116 beats per minute (or 19-29 per 15 seconds).

WHEN AND WHERE TO EXERCISE

Aside from your scheduling needs, you should consider adjusting your daily exercise to the air quality around you--especially if you live in a city or industrial area with harmful toxins like carbon monoxide and sulfur dioxide.

It makes sense to avoid strenuous outside activity during early afternoon when ozone levels tend to peak. If this is not possible, consider joining a health club and doing your sweating inside. If you do stay outdoors, don't do it in the immediate vicinity of heavy traffic.

ALWAYS BEGIN WITH A WARMUP

Every exercise session--aerobic or anaerobic--should begin with a short warmup and then movements designed to gently stretch the muscles you'll be working.

Warming up gradually increases your heart rate, blood flow and muscle action. The stretching phase should be gentle, since severely stretching cold muscles can injure them.

PROBLEMS WITH JOGGING

The jogging craze swept the nation in the late '60s and early '70s, touted as the best of all possible exercises--not only for losing weight and improving fitness, but for cardiovascular health. People who weren't properly prepared for the stress of pounding along city pavements did it anyway, and suffered a catalog of sports injuries--tendinitis, shin splints, bone spurs, etc.

And, in some highly publicized and tragic cases, there were even heart attacks. These usually have resulted when a person suffering coronary disease began a jogging program without medical supervision. In fact, anaerobic exercise of any kind is not usually indicated for people with high blood pressure or advanced cardiovascular disease.

As it turned out, early euphoric claims for jogging did not hold up. Scientific symposiums on jogging have not reported major health benefits. In fact, Dr. Kenneth Cooper, whose aerobic book kicked off the jogging craze, now says that any more than fifteen miles a week gives a person no additional protection from heart disease.

The College of Sports Medicine currently sets its optimal guidelines for running at around two miles a day--which works out to fourteen miles a week, or about the same as Dr. Cooper's recommendation.

Further, most people do not enjoy spending an hour or two running each day--the kind of high-intensity schedule that many jogging-for-your-life regimens recommended. Many others either don't have the time or would prefer to spend leisure hours on something else.

WHAT ABOUT LONG-DISTANCE RUNNING?

There may be other bonuses from long-distance jogging, but increased cardiovascular health apparently isn't one of them. Many joggers, however, speak of the "high" they experience, caused by the brain's natural release of endorphins and enkephalins. And there has been some evidence that marathon running can increase the serum content of HDL, which provides protection against heart attacks. But the evidence is not conclusive, since long-distance runners tend to be in low-risk groups for heart attacks anyway--people who don't smoke, aren't fat, watch their nutrition and so forth.

'PEAK-EFFORT' EXERCISE

Another theory of cardiovascular conditioning holds that a person needs only about ten minutes of peak effort every other day. By doing this (according to Dr. Lawrence E. Morehouse, author of "Total Fitness in 30 Minutes a Week" and formerly director of NASA's manned spaceflight physiology research program), you can reap 80 percent of the conditioning benefits you would get from doing hours of daily exercise.

The point of the peak activity is to raise the heart rate dramatically. The target rate, of course, varies, according to age and physical condition.

WARNING FOR HEART-DISEASE SUFFERERS

People with heart disease definitely need to consult a physician before embarking on any exercise program, especially highly strenuous or peak-output exercise programs.

CAN HIGH-STRESS EXERCISE CAUSE HEART ATTACKS?

You've read the headlines about basketball players, football players, marathon-runners dropping dead. And maybe you wondered, is there a link between high-performance athletics and sudden cardiac arrest?

For instance, on Nov. 29, 1995, two-time gold medalist Sergei Grinkov collapsed suddenly while training at an ice rink in Lake Placid, N.Y He died later that day. The 28-year-old had suffered a fatal heart attack.

Grinkov's death, like the sudden deaths of other famous athletes, has focused attention on a killer that stalks people in the prime of life. Sudden cardiac death kills an estimated 250,000 people in the United States each year, making it a public health problem of enormous magnitude.

One research team, studying this heart hazard, recently identified a genetic flaw that played a role in Grinkov's untimely death. Another concluded that sudden death in athletes can usually be blamed on the heart--specifically, on one of several structural abnormalities.

Grinkov probably suffered no pain on that fateful morning last November. In medical terms, he suddenly went into ventricular fibrillation, a life-threatening quivering of the heart. A medical technician at the ice rink started cardiopulmonary resuscitation, and Grinkov was rushed to the emergency room at the Adirondack Medical Center in Lake Placid.

By the time Grinkov got to the hospital, his heart had stopped. Staff members there nonetheless tried for more than an hour to bring him back to life. An autopsy revealed that Grinkov had suffered from severely clogged coronary arteries.

Although he was an elite athlete, Grinkov had the coronary arteries of a 70-year-old man with atherosclerosis. His widow and skating partner, Ekaterina Gordeeva, told the press that her husband had never complained of chest pain or any other symptoms of heart disease. The only foreshadowing of the impending disaster had been his father's death at age 52 of a sudden heart attack.

Pascal J. Goldschmidt of Johns Hopkins University in Baltimore read an account of Grinkov's death in the New York Times. Goldschmidt, Paul E Bray, and their colleagues had just described a genetic flaw that heightens the risk of early heart attack. He wondered if Grinkov had the trait. So Goldschmidt put in a call to the Adirondack Medical Center. He got lucky: The pathologist had saved a sample of Grinkov's blood and would ship the frozen vial to Baltimore.

When the vial arrived, the Hopkins team first extracted DNA from white cells in the blood sample. Then they searched for a particular version of the platelet antigen gene, which codes for a protein known to play a key role in the blood-clotting process. The group had reported on a link between a variation of this gene and heart attacks in the April 25 New England Journal of Medicine.

Grinkov's blood sample revealed that he, too, had inherited one such gene, presumably from his father. The Hopkins researchers think they know what happened to Grinkov on that fateful day in November. They speculate that a piece of the fatty debris on artery walls broke off and left a hole. But instead of forming just a small clot to plug the injury, a massive clot blocked the entire coronary artery and its flow to the heart.

If future research proves this theory, people with a family history of early heart disease may be able to get a blood test that looks for the gene variant. If they get a positive test, they could take steps to lower their risk. An aspirin a day might be such a step. Aspirin is known to inhibit blood-clotting, so people with a tendency to form clots could take this drug to offset their risk, People with a higher-than-average risk could also cut down on their intake of fatty foods, a factor known to contribute to atherosclerosis.

As previously mentioned, Grinkov was only the most recent champion to collapse suddenly and die. Such deaths have struck athletes ranging from high school team members to professional basketball players.

In the largest investigation of sudden death in athletes to date, cardiologist Barry J. Maron of the Minneapolis Heart Institute Foundation and his colleagues have found that most die from one of several heart abnormalities, only some of which have known genetic links. Most are young athletes who harbor one of these cardiovascular defects from birth, Maron said at a New York press briefing held by the American Medical Association. Such defects "usually cause no symptoms prior to the catastrophe," he added.

Maron and his colleagues detail their findings in the July 17, 1996, Journal of the American Medical Association (JAMA). They collected information on sudden deaths in athletes from 1985 through 1995. The probe turned up 158 such deaths, 134 of them with a cardiovascular origin. The athletes ranged in age from 12 to 40. The largest group, 83 of the 134, was competing in high school sports. However, the series included 16 athletes who had achieved national or international fame in their sport.

Sudden death felled the greatest number of young athletes in basketball and football. It also struck track, soccer, and baseball players and a few in eight other sports. The most common cardiovascular disease identified as responsible for sudden death was an inherited condition known as hypertrophic cardiomyopathy (HCM), a finding in line with previous research.

In this disorder, caused by any one of several mutated genes, the heart's main pumping chamber, the left ventricle, is abnormally thick. The researchers were surprised to find that HCM was responsible for 48 percent of the sudden deaths in black athletes and just 26 percent of the deaths in white athletes.

Other causes of sudden cardiac death in this series include birth defects and other abnormalities of the coronary arteries; aneurysm, or ballooning of the aorta; and myocarditis, a disease that begins with an infection that leads to changes in the heart muscle. A small number of athletes--like Grinkov--suffered from premature clogging of their coronary arteries.

At the press briefing, Maron said that in many cases, physical exertion appeared to trigger sudden death. The researchers found that 90 percent of the athletes collapsed during or immediately after a training session or competition.

How does exertion magnify the risk of a heart attack? That depends on the underlying cardiac condition, Maron says. For people with HCM, strenuous activity increases the chance that the heart will develop arrhythmias, abnormal rhythms that can cause death, Maron points out. For athletes with aneurysms, exertion increases the likelihood that the weakened artery wall will burst. In the JAMA study, only 24 of the 134 athletes had reported symptoms of cardiovascular disease, such as chest pain or fainting spells, in the three years before their fatal episode. Grinkov, who had never complained of chest pain, had apparently been having a heart attack [or hours before he collapsed.

Routine physical exams often don't turn up a cardiac condition in young athletes, that study shows. Of the 134 athletes who complained of heart problems, 115 had received a standard screening. Doctors suspected only 4 of the 115 had cardiovascular disease.

Just one case received a firm diagnosis of a heart condition.

Unfortunately, there's no simple test to detect the variety of cardiovascular ills that may put an athlete in jeopardy, Maron says. "Some are virtually impossible to detect with a routine exam," he says. He favors standardizing the screening process so that more at-risk young people are identified.

Until then, physicians evaluating youngsters for competitive sports must use the tools at hand, including family histories, to find clues to cardiac risk. Indeed, a more aggressive approach to screening might be in order for athletes with a family history of sudden cardiac death, Maron adds. Such athletes may want to consult a cardiologist before signing up for competitive sports.

Heart specialists can more easily detect subtle symptoms of a heart disorder, he adds, A young athlete who does get diagnosed with a cardiac flaw may find the prescription tough to take. For someone with HCM, for example, withdrawal from sports is the only way to reduce the risk, Maron says. Even that course of action is "no guarantee of a normal life expectancy," he adds.

No one knows how many young athletes harbor a silent defect of the heart. Scientists hope that Sergei Grinkov's highly publicized death will leave a lasting legacy in the form of research to improve detection and reduce the risk of sudden cardiac arrest.

WHAT ABOUT WEIGHT TRAINING?

Weight-training comes under the category of anaerobic exercise. But that doesn't mean it can't be part of a total fitness program. In fact, weight-resistance training, also known as strength exercising, offers a number of benefits beyond simply toning or sculpting one's physique. Weight control is one such, but far more important is a measurable decrease in blood pressure. And, as with aerobic exercise, strength training can reduce harmful LDL levels while boosting HDL cholesterol. Blood sugar and insulin levels may also benefit.

In fact, these health advantages are for the taking at any age. In one Tufts University study, people in their eighties and nineties, put on Nautilus machines just twenty minutes three times a week, made almost miraculous improvements.

TREADMILL--BEST CALORIE-BURNER

A recent study of six popular stationary exercise machines came to a startling conclusion: The treadmill, one of the oldest and bulkiest of the home workout contraptions, burns more calories than a stairclimber, a cross-country skiing simulator, a rowing machine and two different cycling machines.

The study, conducted at the Medical College of Wisconsin in Milwaukee, compared energy burned by people using those machines under controlled laboratory conditions at set levels of exercise intensity.

People on the treadmill burned about 40% more calories per hour (705) than they did on the least-calorie-intensive machine, the stationary bicycle (498). In between were the stair-stepping (627) and rowing machines (606), the cross-country skiing simulator (595), and the Airdyne cycling machine (509), which has handles moved by one's arms.

The results go against much popular wisdom, which tends to hold that the more elaborate the exercise machine, the more energy it demands. Many fitness trainers assumed the stair-stepper would finish in first place.

The treadmill's supremacy offers encouragement to people who jog or stroll without benefit of any machine. One obvious inference is that walking and running outdoors or on an indoor track is also going to be a very efficient calorie-burning mode of exercise.

The researchers couldn't entirely explain why treadmill workouts burned more energy than the other workouts. One theory is that running involves many large muscles, from shoulder to toe, working through a wide range of motion.

In contrast, rowing doesn't much involve the large leg muscles, and a stationary bicycle does little from the waist up.

Researchers cautioned that calories burned on a given exercise machine depend on a number of variables, including one's size and fitness. For instance, a large man working out at the "hard" level on the treadmill burned

1,272 calories an hour in the study. A small woman doing the same thing burne only 564.

COMPARING WORKOUTS

The energy expenditures shown below are average values:

Calories per hour

Treadmill: 705

Stair-stepper: 627

Rowing machine: 606

Cross-country ski simulator: 595

Airdyne cycle: 509

Cycling machine: 498

Source: Journal of the American Medical Assn.

TIPS ON USING EXERCISE MACHINES

Whatever home exercise machine you choose, statistics say you'll use it for a very short while, then shove it into a corner or out to the garage and let it collect dust.

In fact, two-thirds of purchasers stop using home equipment after a few intense workouts. Which is about the same as the drop-out rate at health clubs.

Why does this happen? There are several likely factors:

* Many people have unrealistic goals--they overdo at the beginning, don't see immediate results, end up sore and discouraged. These unrealistic dreams are encouraged by "infomercials" which show glamorous exercise professionals and fitness models, instead of people with ordinary bodies.

* Some people aren't cut out to be a successful home-exerciser (where they can be easily distracted) and do better at gyms. One way to recreate that health club environment is to ask family members to encourage or even joinyou.

* Some are suited to home workouts but simply

select the wrong equipment.

* But the majority of dropouts just can't stay motivated.

How to overcome these obstacles: Don't design an entire program aroundthe home machine. For instance, use the stair-stepper or treadmill in thewinter but move outdoors for walking or jogging in spring and summer.

WARNINGS ON HOME EXERCISERS

Exercise riders require considerable knee-bending and hip flexion, so people with joint problems might want to avoid them. Also, overworking hip flexor muscles can contribute to lower-back problems.

Good advice is to consult your doctor before purchasing a rider or anyother piece of fitness equipment, then try it out in the store.

WHAT ABOUT DISABLED PEOPLE?

If for some reason you can't get out andexercise, squeeze your hands into fists. You can do this in bed, in your car,aboard your plane, at your desk, in the john, wheelchair, shower, lunchcounter.

If you can't do this, then you already know you have the exact same blood-serum problem of "settling" that everybody else has. Periodically someone has to turn you. Make sure you get all the right turns during the day, and in most cases, during the night.

If you find you're neglected, complain loudly-- and risk the retaliations. This may be your only exercise. Be sure you get it. When possible, be exercised by a trained therapist or gym coach.

If you've made fists, next spread your fingers, and make fists again.

Do this whether or not you're disabled.

Then turn your hands in circles on your wrists. If possible, point your toes--even seated, you can do this. Then lift your toes. Then circle your foot at the ankle. Keep doing this. Your movement, and your movement only, is what pumps your "lost" blood serum back to your heart. You will feel an immediate pickup.

THE MOST IMPORTANT SINGLE EXERCISE IDEA

Possibly this is the most important single point about exercise for you to know: Your bloodstream is entirely encased in your blood vessels, arteries, veins and capillaries. No blood comes in direct contact with your tissue cells. Your blood communicates, acts and reacts, with your cells solely through the movements of serum.

All of your blood becomes serum, leaving red cells and fibrin behind. At that moment, your blood serum is no longer under pressure, as it becomes the messenger and transport system between your pressurized bloodstream and tissue cells. So far as you are concerned, your serum is lost in your tissues, wandering.

Some of this serum, carrying materials of all kinds, returns to the capillaries, but much of it must be returned to your heart via your immune system, lymphatic vessels and nodes. The speed and health of this fluid are important markers of youth--or age. (When you just sit there, you're not just "resting," you're getting older. When you start to move, you're getting younger.)

WHAT IF YOU DON'T EXERCISE?

The downside is serious. Sedentary folks run twice the risk of heart disease as those who engage in regular aerobicactivity.

The reason is simple. Ongoing aerobic exercise improves heart efficiency.

The heart of an inactive person might normally beat 70 to 75 times per minute,while an active person can pump the same amount of blood while beating only 45 to 50 times per minute--more blood pumped with each stroke. What this means is increased ability to transport life-giving oxygen from the lungs to the heart--and then throughout the body.

Another aspect to this is that exercise tones up the entire musculature,which improves general circulation, reducing the work load of the heart.

Improved circulation means an increase in the total amount of blood moving through the body--more oxygen-carrying red blood cells and hemoglobin, the iron-rich part of the red blood cell.

When oxygen reaches the cells, it combines with blood sugar, or glucose, to cause tiny combustion reactions within the cells. These reactions release the energy the cells need to function.

Unfortunately, according to the Centers for Disease Control and Prevention (CDC), 60% of the U.S. population qualifies as being genuine couch potatoes--a grim statistic responsible for an even grimmer one: 250,000 deaths each year.

As for the lymphatic system, without exercise, when serum builds up in the tissues, the feet swell, the body feels thick, and mood and tone plunge downward. Don't wait "to feel better" before you exercise and pump your own serum and fluids. Begin at once-- you'll feel better very soon.

Your heart serves you quite well. You can do your part and restore the wandering fluids to your heart. It's entirely up to you; indeed, it is up to every human being, every animal on this earth, whether or not he or she is willing to restore this serum to the heart which needs it to become whole blood.Too much resting strains and starves the heart.

All of this advice comes under the heading of exercise--restoring serum to the heart, playing fair with your heart, feeling better, having more fun, getting healthier and more youthful.

That's the deal--any takers?

Notes

_____

_____

_____

VI. ESCAPE FROM STRESS

FEELING STRESSED?

In chapter one we listed the measurable risk factors for heart disease--hypertension, high cholesterol and lipid levels, for starters. These are the factors that medical science has concentrated its efforts on.

Be we also mentioned some unquantifiable (imme surable) risk factors-- negative emotions, like anger and anxiety. We cited a test of more than 2,000 men over more than thirty years, which concluded that anxiety dra- matically increases the risk of both heart disease and of sudden death from all causes.

And medical science has little to say about these things, certainly nothing precise. Only platitudes.

But anxiety can be seen as an outward sign of stress--which has an insidious effect on the heart, blood and blood vessels.

It's hard to isolate since everything in life is a kind of stressor, affecting us in some way--the weather, even pleasant events that accelerate the heartbeat and tense the muscles.

Stress affects people in different ways. Some maintain serenity, while others fly off the handle at the slightest provocation. (Though some outwardly calm individuals may be churning within.)

But scientists are beginning to quantify stress--and see that excessive amounts of it increase the cholesterol in the blood, contributing to atherosclerosis, as well as increasing the heart rate and blood pressure.

So doctors are beginning to join nutritionists and holistic medical experts and therapists and New Agers in realizing the importance of reducing stress, of relaxing.

ABCs OF STRESS

During times of stress two interrelated systems--the autonomic nervous system and the endocrine system--become active.

* The autonomic nervous system controls bodily functions like heartbeat, intestines, salivation and other activities of internal organs.

* The sympathetic nervous system speeds up heart rate, narrows blood vessels, raises blood pressure during physical or emotional stress (a parasymphatetic nervous system works to slow these down when stress has passed).

Related to the nervous system are the endocrine system. The endocrine glands secrete hormones into the bloodstream. This produces various reactions in the organs and body tissues. These hormones are norepinephrine and epinephrine (more commonly known as adrenaline). They stimulate the sympathetic nervous system to raise the blood pressure, continue to increase heart and metabolic rate, and increase respiration to provide more oxygen to muscles. They also increase platelet stickiness, which increases the likelihood of arrhythmias and strokes and coronary artery spasms.

These responses are usually short-lived, designed to deal on an emergency basis with an immediate threat--the old fight-or-flight response to what is perceived as acute danger. Problems occur only when these hormones and reactions continue over a long period of time--this becomes long-term or chronic stress. Here is how this can affect the cardio-vascular system:

* Heartbeat and blood pressure remain elevated;

* Blood sugar is elevated, as are platelet stickiness and serum cholesterol

* Hormones secreted by adrenal glands may injure arterial walls, making atherosclerosis more likely.

* The stress hormones also increase free-radical formation. Remember, these are dangerous molecules that may lead to more LDL cholesterol.

* Chronic muscle tension can rob the body of magnesium and potassium, leaving an excess of calcium and sodium--which can cause abnormal constriction of arteries, including the coronary arteries. And, according to some studies, half of all heart attacks may be caused not by coronary artery blockage but coronary spasm.

HOW YOU GET CHRONIC STRESS

It's not hard, when a typical day may lead you from one stressful crisis to the next, from the alarm clock shrilling to the freeway snarl going home--and the kids yelling and screaming when you walk in the door.

Chronic stress can get another toehold on your internal organs if you try to wind down with smoking or drinking or other high-risk behaviors, like overeating or underexercising.

ASSESSING STRESS

There are three main difficulties in assessing stress:

1. Except for extreme situations, like the death of a loved one or the threat of imminent physical harm, a clear definition of stress is not available. Everything that occurs in your life or exists in the atmosphere is technically a stressor because it affects you in some way. If it is very hot out, for instance, your body will adjust to the increased temperature by cooling the skin with perspiration. In this instance, beat is a stressor because it spurs the body to action. If you receive an unexpected bonus from your boss, the excitement the event stimulates may make your heart beat faster, your muscles tense up, your palms sweat. Despite its positive impact, then, the news of your bonus is a stressor because it forces a physiological reaction-one that will be described in more depth below-to occur.

2. A second problem in relating stress to disease involves how variable our reactions to stress tend to be. Not everyone responds to stress in the same way. Some people become outwardly aggravated over the slightest mishap while others never blink an eye even in the face of disaster. The calm person, however, may be seething inside, perhaps negatively affecting

his or her physiology even more than the person who expresses anger and frustration in a more open way.

3. Even more significantly, stressors vary from person to person. For some, a day spent lying on a beach is completely relaxing, while for others such forced recreation is sheer torture. How you as an individual perceive an event determines how your body reacts to it.

Despite the difficulties in defining and measuring stress, it has become clear that a connection exists between the mind, emotions and health. In the study of heart disease, in particular, evidence has begun to mount that excess stress increases the amount of cholesterol in the blood, thus contributing to the development of atherosclerosis. Stress may also increase the heart rate and raise blood pressure. In many individuals stress results in decreased circulation to the heart muscle itself, often causing the pain known as angina.

Fortunately, it is possible to learn to control both the way you perceive stress and how your body copes with it, at least to a certain extent.

DEADLY EFFECTS OF STRESS

People with a lot of stress in their lives are subject to four basic kinds of reactions, according to many psychologists: physical effects such as body aches, headaches and insomnia; mental problems like memory loss and disorientation; emotional reactions like irritability and depression; and behavior changes that affect interpersonal relationships.

Ultimately, you may become physically ill. You can't shake a flue or a cold, which adds its own stress-

-cutting into your career or relationships. So you may push yourself more and get into a deadly spiral.

What can you do? Glad you asked.

There are proven ways to fight this daily tidal wave of stress--ways to surf these tsunamis and ride them serenely. Take notes. You may save your life.

10 EASY THINGS TO REDUCE STRESS

Here is our short course on stress reduction. It's a mixed-bag of exercise, psychology, attitude-adjustment and sound medical advice. But more than all that, these ten steps are easy and fun. If you don't believe us, try any one of them (or all of them):

1. Shrug your shoulders high, drop them. Gasp for more air, and move shoulders to the front, to the back, to the front. Or just plain jiggle around--move, any old way you can, from head to toe. Shake your legs, bounce.

In other words, work physically on moving lymph. This must be accompanied by deep breathing. Pump the unseen, stagnant lymph through your tissues with as much jostling around as you can get away with. If you're by yourself you can get quite uninhibited, even wild. In the workplace, of course, you may have to close the door, perhaps lock it or go outside and jump around in the park (or parking lot).

Of great advantage here is actually working up a sweat, even briefly. This doesn't have to go as far as a full gym session. That gets out of the "easy" category. But go to the gym if you can.

Note on breathing: Part of the stress response is a tendency to breath shallowly and more rapidly. If you can keep your breathing rate at 12 to 16 respirations per minute instead of 20 or more, you'll be able to short-circuit a typical stress response.

2. After 55 minutes of concentrated work, interrupt yourself. Stand. Or if you've been standing, sit. Make any kind of a change which will momentarily break your chain of thought, your posture and relieve your intensity.

We work ourselves into snarls, mentally and emotionally. Often we go way past the warning signs, the danger signals. We often concentrate so long and so hard that we can bring on harmful conditions. These can be blurred vision, a headache, actually strained muscles.

The greater the stress, and the greater your application to it, the more urgent it is for you to take a break--not just a rest. Not just a stroll across the room. But an interruption.

This is a far deeper matter than appears. If you can, change brain lobes. If you are swarming over pages in a ledger, you're in your left lobe. A real interruption isn't just walking around, it's getting into the other lobe, for even a moment. Enjoy something spacial.

Then finding your way back to the lobe you need for the task at hand will often re-orient you to it, and problems you had before may suddenly be solved.

Call this "lobe-changing."

For instance, if you're in an aesthetic (right lobe) snarl, take a moment to force yourself to do something extremely mundane, practical--find a left-lobe task. You could even sit down and think! If you can, keep it Logical, Linear and Linguistic, the three "L's" of the

Left Lobe. The right lobe is Intuitive, Imaginative and Inspirational.

3. Find something, anything, to laugh about. If you like, collect things for this moment. Reserve jokes, cartoons, stories, gossip--anything that will get a chuckle out of you. Making somebody else laugh is just as good.

Laughter, it has been said, is the king of all medicines. Psychologists have noted for years that many hospitalized mental patients could virtually go home well if they could but deeply laugh or cry. Of course, they can't. That's not just symptom, it's part of the problem.

Our private concerns, you know, are so, so serious! We get to the point where we can't take a joke, and worse, can't laugh--when the belly needs the masterful massaging and jostling of merriment. A single smile, a mere chuckle--these are not true laughter.

Perhaps you read a few years back how the author Norman Cousins literally laughed himself out of a fatal disease by renting some old Marx Brothers movies.

If necessary, collect the things that make you laugh and put them on a spindle so you can't lose them.

4. Have a glass of "perfect" water. Not tap water--unless you've got a perfect filter. Use "natural source"-type mineral water. Or, to distilled water, add a drop or two of liquid minerals (colloidal) from those ancient sea beds which still contain every kind of trace mineral.

We've talked about keeping the blood thin enough to flow easily. Red cells will clump up and block the entrances of capillaries. This cuts off circulation, and proper nourishment is lost.

Again, blood is sticky. The least irritation, wound or irregularity inside an artery can cause platelets to collect. These set off a chemical reaction that starts clotting. Fibrin strands form, and these in turn trap more blood cells--you've got a clot going. And that's dangerous.

Thinning down your blood--without drugs, mind--is a safe, natural, pleasant, inexpensive way to solve these and many other problems. Thick urine and other toxic chemicals can be thinned down by simply drinking a big glass of water. If you can't drink it down, set it nearby and keep sipping at it. It isn't water that overworks your kidneys, it's dehydration.

As a thinning solution, water also helps the kidneys more easily and quickly establish a proper mineral balance. To assist this, a few drops of trace minerals may surprise you. We are, after all, electrical machines, and our electrolyte balance is critical. Minerals are required for electric transmissions in our tissues--and in both the brain and heart. Every heartbeat and every thought is electrical.

Since minerals must be liquefied to be absorbed. At stressful times, this can bring incredible relief--from fatigue, disorientation, confusion, awkwardness, weakness and even numbness in the limbs.

The speed of electrolytic correction can be astounding. I have seen a weak, stumbling person restored to energetic balance in one second flat by drinking a few drops of perfect water.

During stress, huge amounts of nutrition are burned up, and during illness of any kind critical nutrients are lost. Digestive disorders, loss of fluids, traumatic physical injury, tragic news, overfatigue, long-distance running or any extreme physical labor or play--especially during great heat causing heavy perspiration--these are the most prominent causes of electrolyte imbalance, the ones most seriously requiring emergency treatment. But short of such emergencies, just not feeling at your best is occasion enough to drink water and refresh your system. Survival, comfort and diversion--in a single, perfect glass.

5. If you are alone, reach out. Call somebody on the telephone, wave across the way. Go outside and find somebody to ask, "Is this Tuesday?" Or anything--to break the ice, the silence, the aloneness.

Careful surveys touching on thousands of lives have shown that the woman most likely to die of heart attack is the woman alone, who has no deep social or emotional involvements. (The men in their lives may have previouslydeparted via the coronary route.)

Of course, one can be alone in a crowd. I don't know what surveys of men would show, but I expect it would be close to the same. The Greeks said that a man living alone is a bear. Was it the man's clothing they were worried about? His breath? More likely his manners.

Admiral Richard Byrd, famous for his Antarctic explorations and research, lived alone in the blinding whiteness of the South Pole and wrote about it--the loneliness of the white wilderness, no one to look at, no one to laugh with, speak to. It nearly drove him insane.

He said that at certain times, especially right after meals, he would become unbalanced. Part of his misery could have been too much carbohydrate in his diet. This would trigger high insulin. The liver would react, possibly starving the brain, causing clouded thought, confusion.

One day he bolted from his small cabin. There was a blizzard. Before he realized what he'd done, he'd staggered off into the freezing whiteness and, looking around, didn't know which way to turn. If he didn't find the cabin in minutes, he'd be a dead man.

In madness, desperation and the terror of not knowing where to turn or step, he plunged on, searching for that ghost image of his hut--for he could see only inches before his face.

Suddenly, the tiny cabin was there before him. He jerked open the door, stepped inside--and realizzed that, for a while there, he'd been quite mad.

Solitude does this to people. It isn't just the cold or a small habitat. It's the looking up and seeing no one.

Take wise precautions with yourself. Your heart leaps up at the sounds of people you like and their smiling faces.

If worse comes to worse, we believe it would be better for a person to go see someone he or she didn't particularly like than to be always alone.

That is what Admiral Byrd named his book--after the treachery of solitude: Alone.

6. Pet your pet. Or pet someone, anyone--your child, spouse, friend. This could be a simple favor. Hugs are very good. Trust plays a part in this, and that's why pets are perfect--to be petted.

Animals--particularly an animal you like, one that likes you--are the souls of trust. It is that unconditional devotion that lifts up the heart.

Little animals--and not always so little--have a directness, an honesty (even when they're sneaky little creatures) that totally disarms us.

Animals, in grief over a deceased master, have literally languished to death. This is not greed, as some people have said, for a free snack, or remorse over the loss of same. Others have tried to tempt a grieving dog, to feed him or her, to cajole them from their torment.

But then, such animals have frequently been seen to die. You can give your heart to an animal like that. And when stress bears you down, that little creature can offer a kind of affection difficult to find in our more intelligent friends.

In some ways we human beings may have gotten top-heavy. Perhaps that's the reason the crown of the head is denied the honor of wearing the heart, and this symbol of love and life snuggles more modestly unseen within.

It is to this inner recess of private and unquestioning feeling that one ought to bring his little friend, his pet, and find solace, if nowhere else.

7. Go to the mirror and smile at yourself. Self-approval is something everyone is mostly out of. Liking yourself can be very nice--and necessary, especially when one is under stress. People sometimes think this is silly--they'd rather have the stress apparently.

Self-approval, said one noted psychologist, is usually missing when a person says he has faced the truth about himself. We all tell ourselves that we know ourselves best. But the fact is, he said, we are usually too hard on ourselves. Why can we never see that this is unfair?

We evaluate ourselves not in terms of how great we are, but in terms of, first, what we planned to do, and then second, what we failed to do. And this leads to merciless self-castigation.

Just stop all that. Step up to the mirror, and say, "Hi, pal!" Smile. "I'm okay!" "You're okay, we're okay!"

One sales manager told his crew, "I'm not afraid of self-approval. I used to be. Then one day I realized, why, I'm a son of God, and I'm fifteen feet tall!"

That should make you laugh, it's so great. If you don't have a friend to hug, if you don't have a pet to pick up and squeeze and make over, be a friend to yourself--an approving friend--and stop torturing yourself for all your shortcomings.

Your heart doesn't have time for it. Your heart dutifully goes on beating. Give it the same approval you give yourself. Say, "Thank you, you wonderful person! And thank you, my heart--you wonderful heart!"

Gratitude is a heart-filling emotion. And ingratitude toward yourself, denial of your fine points, your rejection of you--all these harm your heart, hurt your heart and give it questionings it should never feel.

Every bad thing you think about yourself reflects upon that fine instrument of life within you. And every good thing you say and think about yourself encourages it, builds it and gives it joy. You can't shame and hurt your heart and help it and please it at the same time.

Your heart doesn't know anything about reverse psychology. So stop injuring your whole vascular system under the guise of modesty. Or worse, unworthiness.

8. Sing! Oh, come on, don't be shy. A bad voice is no excuse. In fact, the worse your voice, the less you sing--right? And the more you need to. Ever hear of good vibes? Well, you can make your own, after all. You don't have to wait for the vibes to come to you, you can emit 'em.

When you least feel like singing is when you most ought to burst into song. Isn't it obvious that "making a joyful sound" is incompatible with stress?

Of course it is. So sing!

When counseling people about their health, we often advise them to sing something every day.

At first, people don't quite believe we're serious. Or they may say that they're not much for singing.

What's wrong with just trying to croak out any old tune? Who cares what it sounds like? Unfortunately, some people are afraid of the sound of their own voices. Singing, somewhere along the line, touches upon the self they've lost.

9. Complete at least one nagging chore. No matter how small it is, do it. But here's the trick: take time to think about why you haven't done this one. Boil it down to the single thing that's stopping you. "Well, I would have sliced that pineapple before it got any older, but--well, I couldn't find the chop board to set it on..."

Then solve the problem. Either find the chop board, or use something else. Don't allow small confusions, tiny frustrations or inadequacies to foil your good intent. After this, enjoy the moment of completion, the deed well done--finally! It's a relief which can turn your whole day around. Call this therapy. It's strengthening.

And remember, stress can be reduced more than one way. Reduce the stress, or get stronger in the face of it. In fact, the second way may be better than the first.

Psychologists have said that no one problem is great enough to break a person. But allow several to accumulate. Add to that an unremitting quality, "These problems, they just won't let up!"

Great deeds, huge steps, remarkable choices, dramatic actions--sometimes these are beyond us. Sometimes we can barely face the day.

That's the time to award yourself a small success. Don't pick your largest stress. Don't grab up a dozen tasks, none of which can be dealt with amply in weeks, even months of time.

No, select some simple thing--but pick one that's been dogging you. Just a little one.

Prove to yourself that you can do it. Draw strength from that one, then try another one.

You can, even in a few minutes, reorient yourself to who is boss and where you stand and what you can do.

They say that the a journey of a thousand miles begins with the first step. Well, your small task, completed and settled, may become for you that first step.

Maybe you can't get the car all shined up. Too many little things interfere. But can you polish one hubcap? Maybe.

What are you conquering? Uncontrol? Yes, but also physical apathy--and all stress aside, its indirect connection to heart disease is fatigued, devitalized blood serum. Slow lymph. Insufficient movement just to be a healthy body.

A healthy body obeys your will better than an unhealthy body.

So start by doing something, and make sure it's small enough that you can succeed--and then look at it. Enjoy your success.

10. Divide big tasks into little ones. Break a hard job into easy steps. If you have six loads of wash to get done, do two this morning. Hold back two for this afternoon. Let the rest wait till tomorrow. This way, it's not such a big deal.

Doing things in stages is easy--unless you're a desperate person who lives in terror of stopping before getting through. (In that case, do all six in a horrendous rush and have your nervous breakdown later.)

Making decisions, many decision in a row, can quickly exhaust the brain. It is said that desk workers burn up as much energy during their day at the office as football stars burn during a hard game.

Still, the brain can restore itself rather quickly if confusion is avoided. Get rid of the confusion and, suddenly, everything seems easy and simple.

Have you seen a person trying to pick up too many articles and dropping several? It's such an obvious mistake, you can see it coming. That's how the brain works, too. Throw too many problems at it in too short a time, and it can get fuzzy, react wrongly, make mistakes, know it, then forget to correct them.

The same tasks can be done with less effort, fewer errors and no pain at all, if taken singly or in small groups which can be solved in short spurts of energy.

The brain is not like an electric drill that can whir through cement, wood and steel. It's not like a clamp or vice that you can bolt onto your workbench and leave fixed for ten years. The brain must, periodically, reach a conclusion. The brain will not readily go forward if there is no light at the end of the tunnel.

So you must be kind to yourself, to your brain, and to your heart: Give your brain short-term goals. You may have, in the back of your mind, the completion of a gigantic job. But you can't do the gigantic job in one brain session--or you'll start dropping things in a clumsy way and only increase your stress.

Instead, apportion your work. When a small portion is done, pause, and briefly survey what remains. Then select the next portion. You can, by easy stages, move through a huge pile of work--and have no, or very little, stress.

This is why businessmen who cannot always clear their desks often make a few neat piles. There may be enough work there, if jumbled together in confusion, to drive a man nuts. But the successful executive sorts through quickly. They deal the papers into piles, tamps them neatly--and have done a favor to their brain, their heart and their life.

Try it. That's the way you talk, isn't it? One word at a time. In little groups called sentences. Paragraphs. Chapters. We can't really comprehend anything else.

No wonder the "anything else's" cause us stress. We must bring such stress into our cognizance, form it into parts and groups and then clear it away.

5 MORE WAYS TO GET A HANDLE ON STRESS

There's no single way to handle all your stresses all the time. And we don't pretend our previous list is all-inclusive. So we've borrowed five more tried-and-true steps toward stress management:

1. Avoid stress or alter the stressors.

For instance, customers' time demands can be very stressful. If you're under too many deadlines, for instance, learn to negotiate with customers for an extension. If you can't get that, consider turning down the job rather than working in high-stress conditions.

Learn to say "no" to others' demands. Hire a short-term employee to help when you're overburdened.

Or, if you're suffering anxiety about being late on making a payment, call the person and explain the situation. Just dialing the phone may be painful, but when you've hung up, you'll have gained at least a temporary resolution of the problem and the stress will be gone.

2. Accept the stress.

There's always some stress in everyone's life. For instance, if you own a business, realize that stress is going to be a part of it. Talking to yourself in a positive way can help you live with it.

3. Talk about the things that cause stress.

Find someone to talk about your problems with. This can be family members, business associates, a support group of some kind, a professional consultant.

The talk can be low-key. A relaxed chat with people who share your perspective will probably offer the best therapy.

4. Exercise.

Every day, if possible, do some kind of aerobic activity. It's a cliche, but absolutely true, when people talk about leaving their problems at the gym. An enjoyable workout is a great stress reliever.

MORE ON FURRY REMEDIES FOR STRESS REDUCTION

Folks with high blood pressure are often told by the physicians to "relax," or "quit worrying."

Easier said than done, right? One stressed-out, high-blood pressure patient had just lost his job, much of his speech ability and control of his muscles, all because of a stroke, or brain attack.

So his doctor came up with an alternative--dogs. "Sometimes the antics and love of a pet can be so entertaining you forget other problems," the doctor said. "Also, the warm body and the unconditional loyalty a dog gives a person is so soothing that it helps overcome stress. This could help to lower your blood pressure."

Shortly after acquiring a white poodle who brightened his life in many ways, this patient went to the doctor for his regular checkup. The result was a significant drop in blood pressure.

Pets have long provided companionship to fill the void in the lives of many people. But health-care professionals are becoming increasingly aware that pets may also help their owners live longer, fuller lives, even after a heart attack or stroke.

This may be because pets, primarily dogs and cats, are non-judgmental sources of affection and companionship. They can create a sense of belonging and responsibility in people who may otherwise feel alone and isolated.

Studies show that in addition to helping reduce blood pressure, pets can help their masters and mistresses lower their heart rate, reduce perceived stress levels and be more active.

"I love pets," says Joseph S. Alpert, M.D., past chairman of the American Heart Association's (AHA) Council on Clinical Cardiology. "Pets are tremendously important as companions for people with heart disease. The more restricted one's life is because of disability, the more important the pet is."

Given the information now available, Alpert says he "endorses the idea--and hopes the AHA will too--that for many patients having a pet is a good idea, particularly when the patient lives alone." He suggests a pet to heart patients, "especially if I think they are depressed or lonely."

Jan Breslow, M.D., president of the AHA, also sees the value of pets for cardiovascular patients. Breslow, who is the Fredrick Henry Leonhardt Professor of Medicine at Rockefeller University in New York City, says studies have consistently shown ways in which animal friends have improved the quality of life for many patients.

Sidney C. Smith Jr., M.D., another past AHA president, recalls his early days in hospital work when he saw the benefits of pets in easing the psychological pain of terminally ill cancer patients.

A professor of medicine and chief of the division of cardiology at the University of North Carolina in Chapel Hill, Smith says, "Social isolation, depression and stress are important factors in the outcome of patients with severe cardiovascular disease. It would be very reasonable to explore the use of pets in this situation."

Smith said lack of social support is emerging as an independent predictor of survival after a heart attack. He encourages studies of the use of pets to provide this social support and to reduce stress in heart patients.

One of the current leaders in pet and social support in the United States is Erika Friedmann, Ph.D., of Brooklyn College in New York City. In the December 1995 issue of the American Journal of Cardiology, she and Sue A. Thomas, Ph.D., R.N., reported on their study of pet ownership and social support in 424 men and women who had had a heart attack and were part of a large study of drugs to suppress irregular heartbeats and prevent a second attack.

When all of the test results were compiled, Friedmann and Thomas found that dog owners are "significantly less likely to die within one year than those who did not own dogs."

Their conclusion was that "pet ownership and social support are significant predictors of survival, independent of the effects of the other psychosocial factors and physiological status. These data confirm and extend previous findings relating pet ownership and social support to survival among patients with coronary artery disease."

Aaron Honori Katcher, M.D., a psychiatrist at the University of Pennsylvania in Philadelphia, and his associates recently set out to examine the idea that animal companionship could significantly increase the survival rates of people with severe coronary artery disease.

Their key finding: Those patients who had a pet had better survival rates than patients without pets. The study makes a strong case for having a pet, which can provide a way to wind down at the end of a tough day.

"Being greeted by your dog or cat when you get home ... can make it all seem worthwhile. A few minutes spent caressing or playing with an animal can be as effective in combating stress ... as a drink or a jog around the block,"

Katcher said in an article, titled "How Pets Aid Health."

Some of the most extensive research on the value of pets has been conducted in Australia at the well-known Baker Medical Research Institute and the Alfred Hospital in Melbourne. When they began their research, Warwick P. Anderson, Ph.D., said he and his colleagues were a "bunch of cynics." So they did a three-year study of 5,741 men and women, ages 20 to 60. They concluded that pet owners had lower blood pressure and blood triglyceride and cholesterol levels than did non-owners.

In a published report, Anderson wrote: "It was impressive for us that all risk factors were lower in pet owners." A total of 784 pet owners took part in the research project; 476 owned dogs and 421 had cats. Other pets included birds, fish, horses and other animals.

The Baker Institute has two other studies underway: an examination of pet ownership in people with and without heart disease and a study of individuals before and after they acquire a pet.

"Last year," Anderson wrote in April 1996 in The Medical Journal of Austral ia, "a comprehensive survey of pet ownership involving 1,011 interviews found that people who owned either a cat or dog visited their doctor less frequently (4.4 times during the y ear on average) than non-owners (5.0 times per year). The pet owners were treated less frequently than non-owners for hypertension (8.6 percent vs. 12.9), hyper-cholesterolemia (2.3 percent vs. 3.5) or for `a heart problem' (3.7 percent vs. 4.9)."

James Lynch, M.D., author of "The Broken Heart: Medical Consequences of Loneliness," and a psychiatrist at the University of Maryland School of Medicine in College Park, is a leading advocate of pets for patients.

"Something as simple as a pet having an effect on health sounds crazy at first, but pets are not irrelevant to people's lives. Lynch's studies have shown that pet owners who suffer non-fatal heart attacks live longer than those who are not pet owners. Pets have other important roles," he says.

"Loneliness is one of the main causes of premature death. Pets serve so many emotional functions. Sigmund Freud once said that the only unambivalent relationship he ever had was with his dog."

While love and companionship are key benefits to pet ownership, pets will never be able to take care of themselves. With ownership come responsibilities and costs for food and veterinary care. All pets need good nutrition and health care. While cats are pretty self-sufficient, someone must make sure they have a clean litter box. In addition, dogs must be walked at least twice a day, and there is also the responsibility of "cleaning up" after the dog. Even the least demanding of all pets, tropical fish, require food and clean, oxygen-rich water.

Do not give someone a pet without first making sure the recipient wants and will care for the animal. Older people or patients may not be "up to" house training a puppy or living with a playful kitten. An older, pre-owned, trained animal may be "just what the doctor ordered."

Remember that acquiring a pet is like adding a person to your life--more responsibility, more work, more pain, but also more fun and more love. For people who want a relatively low-cost, warm and compassionate companion, nothing beats the right pet. And they're good for your heart.

VII. BECOMING A THIN PERSON

HOW MUCH WEIGHT GAIN IS DANGEROUS?

The official definition of "thin" gets thinner all the time. Heart statistics force this upon us.

Why change?

To live longer. And look better.

Overweight is linked to a host of health problems, including heart disease. But at what point is being overweight dangerous?

Two recent studies provide important answers to this question:

The first is the 1976 Nurses' Health Study, which analyzed data from 115,195 women. Researchers found that the risk for dying was highest in the very thinnest and the heaviest women.

However, when the women were separated into two groups on the basis of whether they smoke cigarettes, there was no increased mortality among the very thinnest non-smoking women. But there was a steady increase in risk for dying as weight went up. The heaviest women had four times the risk of dying from cardiovascular disease than the thinnest women.

The second study was of 6,537 middle-aged Japanese American men enrolled in the Honolulu Heart Program. This study also found an increased risk of dying from cardiovascular disease as weight increased.

HEAVY WEIGHT, HEAVY HEART

Because obesity is a major risk factor for cardiovascular disease, weight control has to be a prime objective of any sound nutritional program--and especially one attempting to maximize benefitsfor the heart.

By most reckoning, around 40% of all Americans are not merely overweight but obese, meaning they are 20% above their optimum weight.

Many factors play a part in obesity, of course: Genetics, metabolic differences.

You will find common ground in the opinion that to lose weight, you must burn more calories than you take in.

You will find serious disagreement, however, on what you should eat to boost nutrition and drop pounds.

There have been shelves full of diet books, and more coming out every day. In recent years many of them have concentrated on cutting out fat and adding fiber and carbohydrates. This continues to be the official line in mostmedical journals and books and magazines and TV commercials. But, surprisingly, many of these popular dietary prescriptions will do little or nothing to help you prevent heart attack or lose weight. And the tide is starting to turn, even in popular diet books. And we'll tell you why.

DON'T MAKE YOUR HEART INTO A WEIGHT-LIFTER

Often very heavy people are surprisingly strong. Do you know why? They have to carry so much weight aroundwith them. It takes strong muscles to move a hundred and fifty pounds of fat every time somebody has to trudge to the fridge for supplies.

What's incredible is that so many gorgeous bodies lurk beneath these obese, "Rubenesque" beauties. Those hidden muscles and limbs would look splendid--if we could see them! And if fed properly, those muscles wouldn't shrink and shrivel away with the fat loss.

We've all seen pictures of Opra Winfrey--both ways. Isn't she gorgeous when she takes care to be? And healthier, too. Some of the most famous body-builders carved their physiques down out Michelin-man mass.

BEING A SLIM PERSON IS MORE THAN LOOKS

Consider strength. Often muscles do wither. Crash diets, wrong diets and sheer starvation make the body turn on itself like a starved animal. Self-cannibalization takes place.

You've seen this yourself: a relative goes into the hospital for surgery. Nutrition usually is inadequate, and in three days a strong man or woman is seen to shrink down to a ghost image. Because of this negligence, recovery of millions of patients is slow and too often incomplete. Many never fully recover from the cure.

Why? Because of insufficient protein and other essential nutrients. The body, to stay alive, will digest its own large muscle groups. In the absence of dietary protein, stress forces this cannibalism upon one. For all the incredible cost of hospitalization, most hospitals do not leap into the breach and save the patient such wasting-away. Our wonderful, modern institutions get an F on nutrition.

However, it all goes to illustrate an important point about weight loss: a good diet must not be mere starvation, self-cannibalization, or result in disastrous protein "burning" and weakness. The best diets are those in which the lucky "fat person" gets to eat more than ever! And with three to five medium-sized meals a day, loaded with raw foods which are enzyme-rich and crammed with good fiber for collecting fat--why, we've seen more than one overweight soul complain, "I can't eat all that!"

LOSE FAT, GAIN MUSCLE

If you will increase the right foods, you will correct serious troubles inside. With sufficient protein, your muscle mass not only won't shrink, but may actually strengthen. It has often happened that a young woman's goal of losing fifty pounds was never reached. Oh, she lost fifty pounds of fat, all right, but she gained ten in good, resilient muscle. Why should she be disappointed in this?

With fat loss there will be some slack in the epidermis--loose skin. But consider: if there is muscle loss, too, the skin will sag even more. Your primary defense against sagging skin is to make sure you do not, at the same time, inadvertently lose muscle mass.

DIET THAT FEEDS THE HEART

The real key here is that useful muscles help pump life-giving blood serum and lymphatic fluids back to the heart. Fat does not do this. So the exchange of fifty pounds of fat for ten pounds of muscle is a double gain.

The gain belongs to your heart (and probably to your looks).

The heart no longer is having to support fifty pounds of dead mass (the fat). More serum flows into the heart, nurturing and strengthening it and every cell downstream; while these returning fluids rejoin the red cells abandoned in far-off capillaries.

RETURN OF THE HIGH-PROTEIN DIET

The recent "hot" diet books (according to best-seller lists) promote high-protein, low-carbohydrate eating. In fact, several only tout the glories of high protein while practically banishing bread, pasta and potatoes.

A list of these recent diet books:

* Adele Puhn's "The 5-Day Miracle Diet" (Ballantine)

* Barry Sears' "The Zone" (HarperCollins)

* Richard and Rachel Heller's "Healthy for Life" (Dutton)

* Michael and Mary Dan Eades' "Protein Power" (Bantam)

* Robert Atkins' "Dr. Atkins' New Diet Revolution" (Evans)

All five promise weight loss, increased energy, better athletic performance without hunger cravings.

All of them promote meat-eating again--sometimes in unlimited quantities, like the Eadeses--while warning against carbohydrate consumption.

This advice, of course, flies in the face of the medical establishment. For years, the U.S. government and medical nutritionists have recommended a diet based on six to 11 servings of bread, cereal, rice or pasta; two to four servings of fruit; three to five servings of vegetables; two to three servings of milk, yogurt or cheese; two to three servings of meat, poultry, fish, dried beans, eggs and nuts, and only a small amount of fats, oils and sweets.

However, the prescription doesn't seem to have been working. More and more Americans are overweight. Despite all the low-fat preaching and numerous fat-free foods on the grocery shelves, Americans are getting fatter and heart disease is now again on the rise.

These new diet advisers blame low-fat diets that emphasize carbohydrates. High carb/low-fat eating is wrong and it's making us fatter and prone to disease, believes Barry Sears, Ph.D., author of "The Zone."

Most medical nutritionists insist that the new diets are just like old high-protein diets, especially one pioneered by Dr. Atkins, which have fallen by the wayside. But these new high-protein diets have a new wrinkle: the concept of managing the body's insulin level and keeping the blood-sugar level stable. Carbohydrates, they say, can trigger the body to produce more insulin, which, in turn, encourages it to store more fat.

"Dietary fat doesn't make you fat. It's really the hormone insulin that makes you fat and keeps you fat," believes Dr. Sears. "There are two ways to increase insulin--eat too many carbohydrates or eat too many calories.

Americans do both."

This excess insulin, he explains, sends the body into a fat-storage frenzy. To illustrate his theory, Sears points to the animal kingdom: "The best way to fatten cattle is to feed them lots and lots of low-fat grain. The best way to fatten humans is feed them lots and lots of low-fat grains, as in pasta and bagels."

(For more on insulin and your heart, see "Sugar and Your Heart" below.)

Several of these diets urge patients to eat every few hours, to take moderate amounts of protein, little bread or pasta, and to avoid diet staples, such as low-fat fruit yogurt and bananas, that are high in carbohydrates.

"Protein Power," like Dr. Atkins' high-protein diet of decades past, allows unlimited protein and fat on the theory that people cannot overeat those foods, that they are more apt to binge on high-carbohydrate foods like chips, cookies, cakes and pastries. Dr. Sears' "Zone" disagrees: "There are limits to the amount of protein you should eat. We say you should only eat the protein your body requires. No more, no less."

Protein figures are at a high 30 percent in Dr.

Sears' overall diet, fat is kept to a moderate 30 percent, and carbohydrates are decreased to 40 percent. (Contrast this with some nutritionists' recommendations of 15 percent protein, 10 percent fat and 75 percent carbs.)

Note: A critical part of any weight-loss program, of course, as well as for increasing cardiovascular health, is exercise, as we discussed in Chapter Five.

(**Note:** we'll have more to say about Dr. Barry Sears' "Zone" in the next chapter.)

BONUS FOR THE POCKETBOOK

Fresh, raw foods, vegetables, fruit and bran don't cost as much as meats. We find this both funny and ironic. Fat costs! The fee is less to be slim and healthy!

Have you checked the price of fat-soaked potato chips, lately? And sugared, refined cereals of the most popular kinds? They cost as much as meat!

You can't afford to be fat.

So become a thin person. Just don't "eat yourself alive" doing it.

TRICKING YOUR LIPASE: THE OCCASIONAL BINGE PLAN

There are reasons for deliberately going off your diet. It has been discovered that occasionally, about once every ten days, say, pigging out tricks fat cells into yielding up calories they have been hoarding against famine.

Excessively sudden or extreme diets trigger a strong, defense mechanism of the body. It's exactly as if your fat cells said, "Okay, you gonna starve us? We gonna give you nothin'! We gonna collect and save every tiny, iddy-biddy bit of fat you've got! Okay? Get weak! You gonna starve, you're supposed to get weak!" And that's what happens! Your "health diet" almost puts you to flat on your back.

One good meal, however, and fat cells shout, "Hey! This is more like it! Burn, baby, burn!"--and you begin to burn your own fat more readily for a few days--provided you keep carbohydrates just a little low.

Studies have shown an amazing fact in support of the above comedy: When aroused by sudden fat- or calorie-deprivation, lipase (the body's fat-digesting and fat-collecting enzyme) goes into an orgy of repro-duction--self-replication. So far as this enzyme is con-cerned, you are starving to death. More, not less, fat gets built, because with a sudden saturation of lipase, not one molecule of lipoprotein escapes your tissues.

Alarmed, disappointed, confused, you may desist from your crash diet for a few weeks. But then, your friends make remarks, you see yourself passing in a mirror and disgust finally drives you back to star-vation as the only possible cure.

But guess what? Your fat cells have learned the routine. They're more efficient than ever. The instant you clamp down on them, they start building more fat, and the instant you cease--for more than just one big meal every ten days or so--the fat cells build more than ever.

One crash diet after another is a superb way to teach your fat cells how to build more fat. Want to weigh a ton? Go on one crash diet after another. Your fat cells will soon be smarter than you are! So who's winning here anyhow?

The only solution is a far easier, less starved transition--actually a rather sly transition--to a sensible lifestyle you can live with for the rest of your life. Don't plan just to "get thin." Plan to become a thin person.

COMPUTER DIETING

There are a number of diet programs on the market that can help you keep track of diet and exercise. Life Form (about $40 from Fitnesoft, [800] 607-7637 or [801] 221-7777) is billed as a total health and fitness system that helps track your food and exercise, as well as offering a place to record information about your general state of health, including blood chemistry and history. The program is fairly easy to use and set up.

Heart Smart (Henning Associates, [800] 823-6896) is an inexpensive, also easy-to-use diet program available as "shareware." This means that you can download a free copy from the Internet or an online service or call the publisher for a floppy disk. It costs $19.95 to register. With this product, you can track your calories, fat, sodium, carbohydrates, protein and cholesterol for thousands of foods. Recording what you eat is as easy as dragging the food to your onscreen menu area.

Dieting, of course, is not quite that easy.

WHY NOT JUST USE FEN-PHEN?

Ever since the 1992 publication of a University of

Rochester study, in which Dr. Michael Weintraub combined the two prescription appetite suppressants fenfluramine and phentermine and achieved long-term success, doctors have been taking another look at diet pills. In many parts of the country, fen-phen programs are all the rage. Clinics have even been springing up alongside university-based programs. Family practice physicians, gynecologists and other specialists have incorporated fen-phen programs as profit-boosters. Women make up 80% of fen-phen patients, doctors say.

Some doctors, however, maintain that the drugs are being overprescribed. Lung specialists are concerned about an increased risk of primary pulmonary hypertension, a potentially deadly lung disorder, although the risk to an individual patient may be small.

The most common side effect of fen-phen is dry mouth. Other possible side effects include depression, insomnia, fatigue, diarrhea, blood pressure increases, a feeling of "spaciness" and, in a small fraction of patients, short-term memory loss.

How the drugs work: Phentermine works in the brain--specifically the hypothalamus, is the appetite center--and releases noradrenaline, which lowers appetite.

Fenfluramine raises serotonin levels, decreasing appetite and increasing feelings of fullness. (Increased serotonin generally improves mood, although some fenfluramine users get depressed.)

Dr. Weintraub, now a director of a Food and Drug Administration drug review office, complains that "the medications are being given to the wrong people." He believes that the regimen is suited only for those 30% or more over ideal body weight.

The main problem with fen-phen or any diet pills, however, is that simply decreasing one's appetite does not address maintaining weight loss. For that, a lifestyle change is required--an increase in physical activity and decrease in food intake.

Notes:

VIII. CUTTING CARBS AND SUGARS

THE BODY BURNS CARBOHYDRATES FIRST, THEN FATS

According to Barry Sears and his best-selling "The Zone," it is more the starch than the fat in our diets that builds flab--or at least, the disproportion among the three critical food classes: fat, carbohydrate and protein.

This would be a most difficult concept to buy were it not for the great track record of so many athletes following the regimen; and of course, Sears' rationale.

In simplest terms, his format is not quite a diet, but an easy control of the proportions among those three: fats, proteins and starches:

* Fats--some, but not a lot;

* Carbohydrates--just a little more than protein.

Here's the point: excess carbs turn to sugar. They're supposed to, and must. However, more starch than needed to fuel body cells and the brain at a particular moment causes insulin to mount. This causes the liver (your liver and mine) to cease feeding glycogen back into the bloodstream as glucose. In other words, with heightened insulin, the liver thinks those carbs are "over-sugaring" the blood and cuts off further sugar supplies.

When this happens, with high insulin circulating in the bloodstream, countering glucose and shutting down the liver, there may not be enough glucose in the bloodstream to go around. Because of this, the brain doesn't think as clearly, glands are overworked, and the body goes into a "food drunk" or hypoglycemic spin.

And then, guess what? The body isn't burning available fat.

Why? Because of all that stored glycogen still in the liver, glycogen which can't get out. The body can't switch over to burning fat. In a sense, the body is overloaded and starving at the same time.

Picture the result: a possibly fat person literally covered with potential energy--fat; stuffed with sugar and starch--and not enough energy to move!

At this point, instinctive signals cannot be trusted, for this is exactly when we grab up a candy bar or a doughnut to break the cycle. It appears to break the cycle only because the sugar momentarily overpowers the insulin. But then, even more insulin is injected into the blood to overcome that.

It doesn't have to be that way.

GET OFF THE HYPOGLYCEMIC ROLLER-COASTER

With less carbohydrate in the diet, insulin doesn't rise. Blood sugar may drop, but when it does, the liver will give up its stores of glycogen.

If the liver is slow to react, you can use the mineral, chromium (in edible form, of course) to improve liver efficiency--and then be patient. The lag, as you wait for the liver to come to your rescue, will take less time, day by day. In a few days, a lag of say, thirty minutes may be reduced to twenty minutes. In a few weeks the lag may be no more than two or three minutes. Finally, the day will come when you won't even notice it. There will be no hypoglycemic plunge, and your energy will stay balanced and level.

Then, as the liver yields up its stores of glycogen, turning it into glucose for the bloodstream, and as those stores are exhausted, at that point and only then, does the body switch over to burning its fat.

However, with high carbs, this rarely happens. On the contrary, the "low fat, high-carbohydrate diet" is a formula for getting fatter--as almost every fat-watcher and witness in the country should be able to attest.

In body-building, you will find many athletes following an extremely high carbohydrate diet. Experience suggests that these hi-carbs be taken at least two hours before workout to allow time for the liver to build its stores of glycogen (a solid) from glucose (a liquid). Why? Because this supply really must be converted and burned off as fuel. If not, then we're looking, as always, at more fatty tissue.

Dr. Sears insists that the liver cannot, and ought not, to store enough glycogen to power a heavy workout; and he has shown that muscle mass can best be increased by keeping carbs just a little over protein--with the intention of running out of glycogen, so that fat will be burned instead.

THE CHOLESTEROL-CHROMIUM CONNECTION

Studies indicate that chromium, the trace mineral which helps control the way your body uses sugar and fat, may boost the body's stores of good HDL cholesterol. When people who are marginally chromium-deficient consume more chromium, cholesterol and triglyceride levels benefit, according to clinical trials at the LT.S. Department of Agriculture Human Nutrition Research Center in Beltsville, Md.

Chromium also seems to help those with glucose intolerance avoid developing non-insulin-dependent diabetes. (Having diabetes increases the risk of developing heart disease.)

In another study at Oklahoma State University, 21 people ages 60 and over took 150 micrograms of chromium--three times the minimum recommended daily intake--every day for three months. Another 21 people took a placebo.

Chromium takers with normal cholesterol exhibited no change in their cholesterol levels. But high-cholesterol chromium-takers saw their total cholesterol drop 12 percent and LDL cholesterol 14 percent. Significantly, HDL cholesterol levels weren't affected.

* "Mining" Your Chromium

There's no Daily Value for chromium. But the recommended daily intake of this mineral is 50 to 200 micrograms. The average American male consumes 33 micrograms a day, and the average woman, 25 micrograms.

Good chromium sources include turkey, ham,

grape juice, broccoli, unpeeled apples, green beans and whole-wheat products--and some breakfast cereals. Surprisingly "Total"-brand breakfast cereal is very high in chromium-

-nearly 27 micrograms in one serving.

A more practical chromium solution is a multivita-min/mineral supplement containing 50 to 200 micrograms. Those with diabetes may need even more chromium.

What about side effects? Nutritionists have been studying chromium for decades without a single documented case of a negative effect.

DIGESTION CAN BE A PROBLEM

Carbohydrates--as sugar--are only part of the problem. Complex starches commence to turn into sugars even as we chew them.

That's one of the gifts from our own saliva. And if you don't chew your rolls and cookies and pasta thoroughly, your stomach has to tear them down anyway, or shove them on out, undigested.

All stomachs are not created equal, and while some starch will be digested in the stomach, undigested starch will ferment. Fermentation of this kind actually does cause intoxication. It also can cause esophagal discomfort--gas and burps, interfering with protein digestion to the point that meats then rot, making more toxins. All of which can (and does) overpower not only the stomach, but the pancreas, which is supposed to alkalize the whole mess, overloading the small and large intestines with virtual poison.

BEWARE THE 'STAFF' OF LIFE

Some of these complaints must fall on the starches themselves. Most breads and pastries in this country are produced from intentionally devitalized flours. This means that your body, your heart and your life are robbed when you eat these incomplete foods--even though bread is called the "staff of life." This also depletes you of essential stomach acids, enzymes and hormones.

DIGESTION HAS A PRICE

The cost is internal. We seldom pause to consider that the internal, digestive processing of food, while feeding us, also costs us in terms of our inherent, bodily resources. Too often we use ourmost important molecular and protein structures to digest trash not worth putting through the system.

There seems to be an important, but badly grasped (and certainly denied) quotient between loss and gain. If digesting a sweetroll costs you more than you get--and above all, if it costs you your best resources and gives you back nothing but indigestion and fat--how have you gained?

Answer: You've gained in weight!

You may have enjoyed your brief sugar "high," but all else is a loss. Worse, a lifetime of such empty calories spells heart disease. Researchers are still tabulating the havoc to the body of our "factory-and-materials" wear and tear within; the harm caused by high insulin; the flooding of the bloodstream with excess sugars; the loss of enzymes (which identify food) and hormones messengers (which extract it).

HIGH CARBS: BAD FOR YOUR HEART

Without resorting to an endless list, some aspects of the high-carbohydrate diet must be mentioned here, for the sake of your heart.

Sugar--the destiny of all starches--is always implicated in coronary disease. Need more be said?

Repeatedly, sugar, which damages proteins as well as interfering in our digestion of them, is found to be high dietetically in studies done on who gets heart disease. Further, diabetes (which also means "damaged pancreas") is so frequently accompanied by heart disease that we may say the one goes with the other (though heart disease does not always indicate a damaged pancreas).

The connection, however, of heart disease, sugar and diabetes cannot devolve upon either the heart or the pancreas gland; for the heart and pancreas are supposed to work properly, nothing else interfering. The only thing that's left is--you guessed it--excess sugar. Our eating habits do it to the body, the body doesn't do it to us.

CHOLESTEROL, SUGAR AND YOUR HEART

Sucrose, which is the most common form of sugar, has been linked to higher rates of atherosclerosis and lipid levels, compared with the same calorie diet of starches. A high-sucrose diet is also associated with high insulin levels in the blood. Insulin is the hormone necessary for converting sugar into the body's fuel, glucose. High insulin levels are also involved in arterial wall damage.

More bad things about sugar? It increases the stickiness of platelets. In fact, there is strong evidence that diets high in refined carbohydrates are more associated with heart disease than diets high in cholesterol (see next sections). And high-sugar diets actually promote the excretion of valuable minerals, such as chromium and magnesium.

CHOLESTEROL: NO LONGER THE 'BAD GUY'?

For years it was believed that simply avoiding all cholesterol in the diet would lower blood cholesterol. It happens that cholesterol is found mainly in foods from animals, such as meat, poultry, fish and dairy products. Organ meats, like liver, are especially high in cholesterol. "Plant" foods have zero cholesterol.

But the policy of simply avoiding dietary cholesterol has failed more often than it has succeeded. There are people who have avoided cholesterol religiously for up to forty years, who still have unusually high cholesterol in their bloodstreams.

Now it is known that these people are "cholesterol sensitives" who seem almost to collect it from everything they eat; while others are not "cholesterol sensitives" and either do not absorb it, or quickly discard any excess, and neither show much fat in their bloodstreams nor register elevated pressures.

Individuals interested in protecting their hearts should attempt to learn whether avoidance of this fat in their diet will have any bearing on their health.

There are a number of reasons for this: avoidance certainly doesn't work for everyone. And for others, avoidance is unnecessary. Besides, when anyone becomes too starved for cholesterol, the liver makes more of it. Indeed, every cell in the body has its own store of this oil. Cholesterol is essential to body metabolism. Thus it is foolish to avoid a food which may do you no harm, and which you do actually need.

LEARN YOUR CHOLESTEROL TOLERANCE

For all these reason, it is to your advantage to find out what your cholesterol tolerance is, and control your diet accordingly. And if you cannot tolerate cholesterol--that is, if you tend to "collect" it--this still does not mean that you must give up good food. Rather, there are methods both to lower cholesterol and to relieve elevated pressure, which have nothing to do with avoidance as a way of life.

ANTI-FAT: FACTS AND SUPERSTITIONS

There are certain prejudices regarding various kinds of fat, and these almost amount to superstitions among large numbers of the population. For instance, for at least two decades it was widely held that vegetable oils were far safer than firm, or hard, oils.

Hard fats were condemned. Saturated oils were condemned, unsaturated ones praised. Here's the basic theory:

Diets high in cholesterol and saturated fats can increase blood cholesterol levels. Fats are classified as saturated or unsaturated according to their chemical structure. Saturated fats are derived primarily from meat and dairy products and can raise blood cholesterol levels.

Some vegetable oils made from coconut, palm and cocoa are also high in saturated fats. Most other vegetable oils, however, are high in unsaturated fats. Unlike saturated fats, unsaturated fats, it was believed, do not raise blood cholesterol and can sometimes lower cholesterol.

Unfortunately, some vegetable oils are converted to saturated fats during a process called "hydrogenation" which can be required for food processing.

Unfortunately for these widely publicized and almost religiously believed theories, they do not always square with the scientific evidence, as we shall see. For instance, it has been discovered by ongoing research that reliance on vegetable oils often has produced higher incidence of cancer! But olive and canola oil, which are high in monounsaturated fats, may have a protective effect against coronary heart disease.

Then it was learned that while hard fats, rich in cholesterol, surely can be damaging to the body, they were not always detrimental. For example, hard fats rendered at low temperature do not become rancid nearly so readily or speedily as liquid oils; and further, lard itself tends to build HDL more often than LDL.

CHOLESTEROL-FIGHTING NECTAR

Olive oil was prescribed as a natural remedy more than 2,000 years ago no less a physician than the great Hippocrates. It wasn't superstition. The fragrant oil is full of monounsaturated fat, which tends to trim LDL cholesterol while boosting HDL cholesterol.

One study suggests that olive oil may actually change the chemical composition of HDL cholesterol, improving its ability to combat LDL. With this kind of potential benefit, some heart experts have recommended substituting olive oil for all other kinds of dietary oil.

Of course, too much of any fat--even monounsaturated--can pump up your cholesterol level, and your belt size. Olive oil is still 100 percent fat and contains 120 calories per tablespoon, so overusing it may cause you to gain weight. But you don't need a lot of olive oil. A little bit yields considerable flavor. And the golden fluid tastes great on everything from corn to crusty bread.

The so-called Mediterranean "miracle" was first documented by Ancel Keys, Ph.D., professor emeritus of public health in the School of Public Health at the University of Minnesota in Minneapolis. In the 1950s Keys noted that while Italian, Greek and other Mediterranean men consumed almost as much dietary fat as Americans, most of that fat was in the form of olive oil. He associated the Mediterraneans' consumption of monounsaturated fat, particularly olive oil, with their lower rates of heart disease.

More recent studies--at the University of Madrid and again at the University of Nijmegen in the Netherlands--have reached similar conclusions.

OLIVE OIL BASICS

Connoisseurs categorize the flavor of olive oil as mild (a light or buttery taste), semifruity (stronger, more olivelike flavor) or fruity (an intense olive flavor).

The color of the oil, however, has nothing to do with its flavor. Like wine, olive oil gets its unique color, flavor and aroma from the olives used and the climate and soil conditions in which they were grown. Taste-test oils to find the variety and brand you like best.

How to get more olive oil into your diet:

1. Spread crusty bread with olive oil rather than butter.

2. Dress salads with a small amount of extra-virgin olive oil and a little bit of vinegar.

3. Brush corn on the cob with extra-virgin olive oil rather than butter or margarine.

4. Add olive oil to sauces, marinades and any other dish in which you want a stronger flavor.

5. Bake with olive oil. You can substitute olive oil for butter, margarine or vegetable shortening in cakes, pies and other desserts. A light variety is recommended so the olive oil taste doesn't overpower the dessert.

(**Note:** Heating extra-virgin olive oil is not recommended, as it goes into the air rather than into the food. Save extra-virgin for salads or for drizzling over pasta.)

Here's a guide to help you decipher olive oil labels:

* Extra-virgin: Produced in limited quantities, extra-virgin oil is the best and most expensive grade. Extra-virgin oil has an intense fruity or peppery flavor, and can be used to flavor foods after they've been cooked rather than as a cooking oil.

* Virgin: The flavor isn't as perfect as that of extra-virgin and is slightly more acidic.

* Olive oil: The blend most people use for cooking.

"Light": Perfect for baking, this extra-refined oil has little or no olive taste. Note: Light olive oil contains the same amount of fat and calories as other oils.

AVOCADO: FAT-FIGHTING FRUIT

Avocados, a fruit which many of us mistake for a vegetable, are high in monounsaturated fat and especially rich in oleic acid, the cholesterol-reducing monounsaturate found in olive and canola oils.

The catch: Avocados are high in fat. But eaten in moderation, they might help you pare a few points off your cholesterol count.

The link between avocados and blood cholesterol was discovered by Australian researchers. They had 15 wo-men alternate between a low-fat, high-carbohydrate diet (21 percent fat calories) and an avocado-enriched diet (36 percent fat calories).

After three weeks on the avocado-rich diet (from 1/2 to 1 1/2 avocados per day) the women's total cholesterol fell from an average of 8.2 percent, compared with 4.9 percent after three weeks on the low-fat plan. Even better, while the "good" HDL cholesterol actually dropped an average of 14 percent on the low-fat plan, there was no drop at all on the avocado diet.

Avocados may be especially prescribed for people with non-insulin-dependent diabetes, for whom consuming too many carbohydrates can cause triglyceride and blood sugar problems. Partially replacing carbohydrates withmonounsaturated fat has been found to lower triglycerides in women with this type diabetes.

From 71 to 88 percent of the avocado's calories come from fat. The trick is to substitute avocados for foods high in saturated fat rather than add avocados to an already high-fat diet. Most people don't eat more than half an avocado at a time, usually adding chunks or slices to salads or a sandwich. Here are other serving suggestions:

* Top baked potato with mashed avocado.

* Top baked chicken with slices of avocado before serving.

* Add mashed avocado to potato salad.

* Slice an avocado in half, remove the seed and stuff the fruit with chicken, seafood or pasta salad. To keep the avocado from turning brown, rub the flesh with a little lemon juice.

Note: If you buy avocados not yet ripe enough to eat, speed up the ripening process by putting them in a paper bag and setting them aside a few days.

OLESTRA: IS THE NEW 'FAKE FAT' SAFE?

Early this year, the U.S. government approved the use of olestra, a calorie-free fat substitute hailed by its manufacturer as a boon to the overweight. However, it has also been characterized as a danger to the public's health.

Unlike other fat substitutes, olestra can withstand the hot temperatures necessary for deep frying and is therefore suitable for use in savory snacks. Because of its chemical makeup, this "fake fat" is undigestible and passes through the body without being absorbed. In this way, the pleasing flavor and texture of the food are retained but no fat or calories are added.

The approval by the Food and Drug Administration (FDA) specifies that olestra can be used in snack foods such as potato chips, tortilla chips, cheese puffs, and club crackers. Procter & Gamble will market the product as

Olean and sell it to makers of snacks and crackers. Use of the product in other types of foods would require additional FDA approvals. Test-marketing of products containing this fake fat began in the spring of 1996.

* Possible downside

You'd suppose that overweight folks should welcome olestra as a painless way to reduce calorie consumption. But many experts encourage caution.

Why? Because olestra brings with it potentially harmful nutritional and gastrointestinal side effects. Even in low doses, this artificial fat inhibits the body's absorption of the fat-soluble vitamins A, D, E, and K. Olestra also reduces the absorption of some carotenoids--nutrients found in carrots, sweet potatoes and green leaf vegetables.

In one study, even the daily consumption of a small amount of olestra--less than that found in a small snack bag of potato chips--reduced blood levels of one carot-enoid, beta carotene, by 60%. Many epidemiological investigations have shown that low intake of carotenoids--or low blood levels of them--are associated with an in-creased risk of coronary artery disease, stroke, many cancers, and eye disease.

Malabsorption of the fat-soluble vitamins has the potential to cause other problems. Older people--particularly if they are housebound and get too little sun--may not take in enough vitamin D, which can help prevent osteoporosis. Variations in the levels of vitamin K, which promotes blood clotting, might alter the effect of anticoagulants in people with bleeding disorders.

To offset the effects of vitamin loss, Olean will be fortified with vitamins A, D, E, and K. But does "fortification" and "replacement' of these vitamins furnish them in a way that they can be absorbed normally?

Will the vitamins added to olestra be absorbed by people who eat foods containing the fake fat? Or will the fat substitute, even though fortified, still draw vitamins from the other foods in a person's stomach and carry them out of the body?

In addition to the malabsorption problem, olestra can cause intestinal cramps and diarrhea. Therefore, the FDA is requiring that all products made with olestra have a warning label and has suggested: "This product contains olestra. Olestra may cause abdominal cramping and loose stools. Olestra inhibits the absorption of some vitamins and other nutrients. Vitamin A, D, E, and K have been added." The specific words of the final warning label will be determined by negotiations between the FDA and the manufacturer.

* Weight loss and olestra

What about the weight loss anticipated by people who consume products made with olestra? There is no proof that olestra helps people slim down, and experience with sugar substitutes suggests that people may very well gain weight on olestra. For instance, in the famous Nurses' Health Study, the single best dietary predictor of weight gain was saccharin consumption. In another study, people who used artificial sweeteners were on average two pounds heavier than people who did not. The prospect of eating snack foods containing olestra may actually encourage people to eat more than they might otherwise.

In general, people who eat snack foods are unlikely to stop at eating one ounce--the amount used in some of the research conducted by Procter and Gamble. A one-ounce serving of potato chips contains about 10 to 15 chips.

People who purchase a bag of chips at the grocery store are more likely to buy at least a five-ounce bag.

* Long-term safety

Critics of olestra point out that the studies presented as evidence of olestra's safety were sponsored by Procter & Gamble. Furthermore, these critics maintain that all of the studies have been small and short-term. These scientists contend that the studies were inadequate to demonstrate long-term safety and that there have been no demonstrated benefits in weight reduction due to olestra. Still other critics are concerned about the effects olestra will have on children.

As a condition of approval, Procter & Gamble will conduct studies on olestra's long-term effects, and the FDA will formally review these studies in a public meeting of the Food Advisory Committee held by July 1998.

Conclusion: It makes more sense to avoid unhealthy fats the old-fashioned way--by just not eating them--rather than by consuming products that contain olestra. More to the point, most Americans already fail to consume enough of vitamins A, D, E, and K because they eat too few fruits and vegetables.

And the fat-soluble vitamins A, D, E, and K and carotenoids need real fat for their absorption. Olestra actually inhibits this process.

A HEFTY DEFENSE OF LARD

Some nutritionists consider lard the most misunderstood of fats. According to the USDA it has less than half as much cholesterol as butter. On the other hand, it contains a large amount of oleic acid, which actually helps break down cholesterol.

Considering lard's current disrepute, it's difficult to believe that up until the '20s, before most commercial oils and shortenings, lard was the principal cooking fat in the United States. In fact, when vegetable shortening came on the market, Crisco tried to look as much like lard as possible.

An obvious factor in lard's fall from popularity, of course, has been the discovery of the connection between cholesterol and animal fats such as lard, butter and beef tallow. But fats and oils, which differ mainly in that fats are solid at room temperature, have more in common chemically than people think. Both are made up of a glycerol molecule linked with three compounds belonging to the group known as the fatty acids.

A fatty acid molecule is a chain of carbon, oxygen and hydrogen atoms. The length of this hydrocarbon chain varies, but there is a maximum number of hydrogen atoms it can have. If a molecule has its full capacity of hydrogen, it is called saturated. If it has two fewer hydrogen atoms, it's mono-unsaturated, and if it has room for four or more hydrogen atoms it's polyunsaturated.

Though shortening and margarine are made from plant sources, they have to be hydrogenated (saturated) to gain a solid consistency. The hydrogenation process also produces trans-fatty acids, which are considered to be as harmful as saturated fats in causing coronary heart disease.

The hydrogenation process also lowers the smoke point (the temperature at which fats break down into gas). Smoking margarine or shortening doesn't just smell bad, it produces chemically active materials that remain in the liquid and may ruin the flavor of fried foods. And the scorching also produces the chemicals classed as free radicals, which have been associated with cancer.

FIGHTING THE FAT-IN-FOOD PROPAGANDIST

The topic of cholesterol has become one of contradiction, confusion, possibly leading to increased, rather than de-creased, illness. And, without any doubt, the ensuing fears have ushered in an overall loss in eating pleasure--which also doesn't contribute to health.

One pat of butter will not give you a heart attack. But long years of inactivity and poor diet, as well as stress (all by itself) can bring on many heart diseases and ultimately death.

Dr. Linus Pauling was one of the first to speak out against the conventional medical "wisdom" that reducing dietary cholesterol is the panacea for heart disease. He cited the 1970 Framingham study of diet in relation to heart disease that confirmed that restricting the intake of cholesterol does not reduce the cholesterol level in the blood.

As Dr. Pauling pointed out, human beings synthesize cholesterol in their own cells and decrease the rate of synthesis when the cholesterol intake is increased. There is no reason for people to deprive themselves of a reasonable amount, therefore, of such good food as eggs, meat and butter.

By the mid-'80s, it was quite obvious to Pauling and others that the great hope that heart disease could be controlled by limiting the intake of saturated fat and cholesterol and increasing unsaturated fat, especially polyunsaturated fat, had failed abysmally.

And yet, foundations and scientists and the media have continued to this day to trumpet low-fat, low-cholesterol, polyunsaturated diets, while the epidemic of coronary disease has continued unabated. These anti-fat propagandists are doing so in the face of overwhelming clinical evidence--study after study showing that reductions in the amount of dietary cholesterol have no significant effect on the incidence of heart disease.

SUGAR INTAKE AND CORONARY DISEASE

As we've said, absolutely no correlation has been found between the intake of fat and the incidence of heart disease--despite the continued trumpeting of this myth. There actually is far more clinical evidence of a link between coronary disease and the intake of sugar. The other half of that link is that sugar intake increases blood cholesterol.

(Excessive amounts of sugar and alcohol can also drive triglyceride counts way up. And too often cholesterol-watchers, told to avoid fats, turn to sugar-laden foods.)

One study in 1957 compared death rates from coronary disease in fifteen countries to the average sugar intake. The annual coronary death rate per 100,000 people rose steadily from 60 for an annual intake of 20 pounds o sugar to 300 deaths for 120 pounds per year. There have been many followup studies confirming this linkage.

There is confirming evidence, as well, from another discipline--medical history. Coronary disease is really a modern phenomenon, as we stated in our introduction. We find almost no references to it beyond the last hundred years--the period during which we have begun consuming vast amounts of refined sugar.

There are many primitive populations with diets high in animal fat, and all of them report very little heart disease. When those populations become urbanized, however, and begin consuming sugar, the incidence of coronary disease rises rapidly.

The average American gets 20 percent of food energy from sucrose, which works out to around 125 grams of sugar per day, or 100 pounds a year--far beyond what is safe, let alone healthful.

CALCIUM VS. SUGAR

Table sugar is the simple carbohydrate, sucrose, which is a combination of glucose and fructose. Their molecules have some similarities to those of calcium--a very unfortunate state of affairs for human health.

Now, in our mind's eye, let us look inside the

heart.

The myocardium is the middle layer of the walls of the heart and is cardiac muscle. It is the seat or surrounding "fist" containing right and left ventricles.

When the myocardium contracts, it forces blood to leave the heart, surge into the lungs, return into the heart again and then stream out through the upper and lower arteries, upon its way to nurture and restore the entire body. The miraculous agency which causes this muscle to contract and therein create the tremendous pressure necessary to push blood through those incredible sixty-thousand miles of blood vessels is electricity.

Calcium, among other nutrients, is stored in your myocardium and participates in the electrical firing of every beat of your heart, your whole life long. This mineral, calcium (as just one example of many such nutrients), not only enables the heart to beat but eases the heart during sleep, is a pain-killer and a mild sedative.

You need calcium in your myocardium. But sugar not only resembles calcium in some ways, it is antagonistic to calcium. Sugar literally dissolves teeth. Indeed, sugar plays havoc whenever it and calcium meet, as if contesting for the same ground. Often, tragically, sugar wins.

Worse and worse: Sugar does not transport electricity, is not a mineral, damages proteins and does not build cells, even if it feeds them. Sugar cannot replace calcium, but it can, and does, displace calcium.

You must have calcium in your bloodstream, not only to build strong cell walls, but to make the heart muscle contract--and relax. Sugar, while antagonistic to calcium, performs none of calcium's vital functions.

Sugar is a food, a fuel, not a structural element. Thus, the least overabundance of sugar, where calcium is at work, spells disaster.

DANGERS OF EXCESS SUGAR

Sugars of certain kinds are essential to life and especially to the feeding of the brain. But sugar above necessary amounts is clearly not just a minor poison. In elevating insulin above normal it makes the brain groggy, stupefies the sensibilities, makes children hyperactive andall but crazy; it feeds herpes simplex and other viruses, thereby lowering immunity disastrously.

Thus the least amount of excess sugar becomes, both in the bloodstream and via the pancreas as high insulin, a lunatic impostor-"nutrient" and a downright killer.

A diet low in calcium and high in starch, carbohydrate and sugar will show every disorder from hypoglycemia to a damaged pancreas, pre-diabetes and eventually heart disease, to say nothing of rotting teeth, acne, increased virus presence and a troubled disposition. You cannot build calcium structures, heart muscle, teeth and bones, or strong cell walls (or good, sound sleep) with calcium's look-alike but evil twin: sugar.

SUGAR `TAKES THE CAKE'

Did you know that many commercial cake-frostings, which look like sugar, taste like sugar and "set up" like sugar, began as oils? That is, fat--primarily animal-source lard. And frequently rancid fat to boot? Fat can be turned into sugar. Tar and crude oil can be turned into sugar. Likewise, your body can turn fat-to-sugar right back into fat. And if you have unused sugar in your liver, you'll never burn remote fats away.

Why does this pose a problem? Because the real bandit in diabetes (and, thus, heart disease) isn't sugar only, but its close associate, fat.

Such disquieting facts are usually ignored. Yet sugars can and do turn into fat. Fat is implicated in diabetes more than sugar itself. Diabetes is accompanied by heart disease. Therefore, sugar above the essential, absolute minimum is a heart-damaging food.

Let's say this again: excess carbohydrates and the ensuing sugars which habitually raise insulin levels prevent the burning of carbohydrate stores; this in turn prevents the burning of body fat.

If repeated supplies of carbohydrate keep insulin high, the unused sugars will be turned into more fat.

Until this self-destructive cycle of utterly misleading "high-carb and (supposedly) low-fat" diet is interrupted, the excess, unhealthy bodyfat will stay in place, right where it is virtually forever. This fat will not be burned away or used for its rightful purpose--as energy.

HOW TO CUT YOUR SUGAR 'FIX' IN HALF

It's not that difficult to decrease your intake of sucrose, and the benefits are well worth the discipline. Here are four guidelines:

1. Get rid of the sugar bowl entirely. One heaping tsp. of sugar weighs 9 grams. That's a significant amount to avoid. Which means you should eat sugar-free cereals (not frosted), and then add only a very small amount of sugar to them (if you must).

2. Avoid sweet desserts--if possible. The common sources of sugar in the American diet (besides soft drinks) are snacks such as jams and jellies, ices and ice creams, gelatin desserts, syrups and pastries.

3. Avoid sweet snacks--jellies, jams, ices, gelatin.

4. Stay away from soft drinks (except carbonated waters). One 6-oz. can or bottle of cola contains 17 grams of sucrose. Four of those a day equals 155 pounds per year.

What about diet sodas? There are various opinions on artificial sweeteners. But many nutritionists remain concerned that these substances may have toxicity.

WEANING YOURSELF FROM STARCHES AND SWEETS

Here's another trick, if you're really serious about reducing bodyfat, for weaning yourself away from starches and sugars and sweets. Try this:

When eating out, ask for a few slices of lemon. Squeeze the lemon slices into your drinking water. Toss the rind in, too. Don't add one grit of sugar.

You will have a refreshing drink, the water will have flavor. And you will have begun teaching your taste-sense to go toward the sour--which the stomach loves--away from the starchy and sweet. After lunch, brush your teeth.

Or this:

Purchase ascorbic-acid crystals. That's vitamin C in crystal or powder form. (For this purpose, avoid calcium-ascorbate, which is still useful, but not for this purpose; it doesn't taste so good.) Add pinches of the straight C to most your food and drink.

Careful, here. Pure C is very sour--but that's what you're after.

For instance, add 1/8th teaspoon of C crystals (about 250 milligrams) to a quart of drinking water and store in the refrigerator for cool drinking.

Let one pint of ice cream come to room temperature. Stir in the juice of half a lemon and 1/4th teaspoon C crystals--that's a whole gram (1,000 milligrams). The ice cream will not be sickeningly sweet and will, for that reason alone, taste better. Whip the balance, repack into the container and store.

And once again, brush your teeth.

You will soon learn that all sweetened foods are really far too sweet.

You can begin to defeat the cravings for such things right there in the mouth where these delicious sugar-crimes are committed.

Your taste buds can easily be brought under the spell of your imagination. They will learn to do exactly what you tell them, show them and teach them--if you will make the attempt.

It's a small turnaround. Instead of your imagination being enthralled with your mouth, make your mouth the servant of a rational and advised imagination. Use real and simple flavors to do this.

We know many people (including ourselves) who used to be sugar-freaks.

Today they can hardly stand to have, for example, candy in their mouth, only accept it to be polite, then turn away and inconspicuously spit it out.

You can get to the point where you simply won't enjoy most fattening pastries and will think, "This is just more flab I'll have to get rid of."

You can learn what these annoying, non-foods really are--and aren't.

As the mists of illusion and childish teething evaporate, your desires will turn to foods really good for you. And you'll find that your pleasure in eating them, their flavor, their taste, corresponds to their real value.

Notes:

_____

_____

_____

_____

_____

_____

IX. THE WONDERS OF BRAN AND WATER

WHY FIBER IS GOOD FOR YOU

A few years back, oat bran grabbed all the headlines as a weapon against heart disease. Since then, the spotlight has been turned on garlic, red wine, olive oil and various vitamins. But it's high time we took another look at bran, and why it needs to be part of your daily intake.

Say "fiber" or "bran" and you may think "laxative." Indeed, bran is well known for its bulking effect and for keeping food moving in the digestive tract. But fiber's power to unclog your backed-up plumbing is only part of the story. Numerous studies suggest fiber can help unplug arteries, too, lowering elevated cholesterol. So the main purpose for listing this old saw at this point is something else entirely: some kinds of bran collect fat.

By "bran" we mean primarily:

A. Oat bran.

B. Psyllium.

C. Guar gum.

These offbeat foods should become staples--in small amounts.

You don't need to eat a lot of them, but you must ingest them with food, especially with the "fatty" ones in question. Recent research has demonstrated beyond doubt that these simple remedies, taken between meals, have no effect upon cholesterol. That is, without direct contact with the food.

These dramatically effective, peculiar, husklike foods must come in contact with foods eaten at meals or with snacks to reach the cholesterol you wish to get rid of.

PAINLESS WAY TO 'EAT YOUR OATS'

There are two basic types of fiber: soluble and insoluble. Soluble fibers such as pectin, psyllium and guar gum, found in foods such as oat bran, barley, dried beans, peas and apples, seem to help control the way your body produces and eliminates cholesterol.

Soluble fiber helps lower serum cholesterol, according to many recent cliinical tests. Insoluble fiber, abundant in whole-grain products, fruits, vegetables and cereals, is the stuff that helps keep you regular, speeding food through the system and bulking up your stool.

Our suggestion is that you get these fibers down mid-meal. You can find them in capsule form for convenience, travel and simplicity when too rushed to stop and stir.

Because they are water-soluble and form a kind of gel in the stomach, these fibers trap cholesterol. Be sure, at this time, to enjoy some extra water--that is, extra good water. Dry, these fibers are not active and no gel forms.

As little as 2 level (or 1 rounded) teaspoonsful of oat bran taken with sufficient water to make the "gel" helps to carry cholesterol from your body.

As this happens, everything else higher up in your body is relieved of stress, including your heart.

Bran detoxifies the intestines and colon, gradually buffing dead cells, decayed matter and foreign substances from intestinal walls, bulking difficult foods, and above all, collecting fat in the mesh created by soluble bran fibers and gel.

Scientists have conducted numerous studies of fiber's power to reduce cholesterol. In one study at the University of Kentucky College of Medicine in

Lexington, researchers divided 146 people with moderately elevated cholesterol into three groups. The first group ate their usual diets. The second group followed a low-fat diet that contained 15 grams (about a half-ounce) of fiber.

The third group consumed a low-fat diet packed with 25 grams of fiber.

After a year, the low-fat, high-fiber group's total cholesterol had fallen 13 percent, compared with a 9 percent drop in cholesterol for the low-fat group and a 7 percent decrease in the folks who ate their usual diets.

Researchers noted that the fiber boost came from common foods easily added to an ordinary diet--one bowl of cooked oat bran cereal, two small bowls of cooked oatmeal or about five ounces of canned beans a day.

In another study, researchers at Stanford University School of Medicine had 16 people consume 15 grams of soluble fiber (including pectin and psyllium) a day. These volunteers' total cholesterol fell 8.3 percent, while their "bad" LDL cholesterol dropped 12.4 percent, in just one month.

So eat your brans religiously.

'FIBER UP'

The simple formula is: If it crunches, eat it. Fact is, most of us consume less fiber than we should--less than a half-ounce) a day for most

Americans, instead of the 25 to 30 grams we need. But it's easy to "beef up" your fiber intake. Here are some tips:

* Eat the skins of fruits and vegetables (such as apples and potatoes) as well as fruits with edible seeds, like figs and blueberries.

* Don't depend on a high-fiber cereal whose manufacturer claims that you can get all of your fiber in one bowl.

* Drink eight to ten glasses of water a day. As mentioned earlier, fiber absorbs fluid as it passes through the body; not drinking enough water can lead to constipation.

* To minimize gas and bloating--common side effects of consuming more fiber--add fiber-rich foods to your diet slowly.

* Take bran in capsule form--any one or combination of this group of three basic "brans," oat bran, psyllium or guar gum. At mealtime it's simple, quick and unobtrusive.

DIETARY SOURCES OF SOLUBLE FIBER

Want to crunch down on high cholesterol? Try these high-soluble-fiber foods.

FOOD	Total Fiber (g)	Soluble Fiber (g)
All-Bran cereal (1/3 c)	8.6	1.4
Apple, with skin (1 small)	2.8	1
Barley, raw (2 Tbsp.)	3	0.9
Blackberries (1/4 c)	3.7	1.1
Blueberries (3/4 c)	1.4	0.3
Brussels sprouts (I c)	5	2.6
Carrot, raw (1)	2.3	1.1
Chick-peas (1/2 c)	4.3	1.3
Corn bran, raw (2 Tbsp.)	7.7	0.1
Figs, dried (3)	4.6	2.2
Grapefruit, pink (1)	1.4	0.3
Honeydew, cubed (1 c)	0.9	0.3
Kidney beans, cooked (1/2 c)	6.9	2.8
Lentils, boiled (1/2 c)	5.2	0.6
Lima beans, canned (1/2 c)	4.3	1.1
Oat bran, dry (/3 c)	4	2
Okra (1 cup)	7.3	2.9
Orange (1 small)	2.9	1.8
Pear (1 small)	2.9	1.1
Peas, frozen, cooked (1/2 c)	4.3	1.3
Pinto beans, cooked (/2 c)	5.9	1.9
Plums, red, with skin (2 medium)	2.4	1.1

Potato, baked (1)	5	1.2
Pumpernickel bread (1 slice)	2.7	1.2
Raisins, seedless (1/2 c)	1.6	0.8
Spaghetti, whole-wheat, cooked (1 c)	5.4	1.2
Spinach, boiled (1/2 c)	1.6	0.5
Sweet potato, baked (1)	2.7	1.2
Turnips, cooked (1/2 c)	4.8	1.7
Wheat germ, toasted (/4 c)	5.2	0.8
White/navy beans, cooked (1/2 c)	6.5	2.2

MORE ON THE POWERS OF PSYLLIUM

There's even more evidence that this natural laxative can help lower blood cholesterol.

Several studies have shown that psyllium can reduce moderately elevated blood cholesterol. That's because psyllium, derived from the seed husks of a plant with origins in India, is rich in soluble fiber, a gummy substance found in certain fruits and vegetables that has been shown to deflate cholesterol.

As previously mentioned, psyllium is available in supplement form, such as powders and wafers, as well as in some breakfast cereals.

How it works:

Studies suggest, that like other forms of soluble fiber, psylliumprevents the body from reabsorbing a digestive secretion called bile. If there is soluble fiber in the small intestine, bile--which contains cholesterol--gets trapped in this gummy substance and is excreted from the body. Without soluble filter, the body reabsorbs bile and recycles its cholesterol.

In one University of Kentucky clinical trial, 44 people followed a low-fat, low-cholesterol diet. They ate either a psyllium-enriched breakfast cereal or a wheat bran cereal containing negligible amounts of soluble fiber.

After six weeks, LDL cholesterol dropped nearly 13 percent in the people who ate the psyllium-enriched cereal but only 2.5 percent in the wheat bran group.

These results were reinforced by research at the University of Cincinnati and Washington University School of Medicine in St. Louis. One-hundred eighteen people with elevated cholesterol (220 milligrams/deciliter or higher) were placed on either a low-fat or a high-fat diet. Some consumed five grams of psyllium (in sugar-free orange-flavored Metamucil) twice a day, just before breakfast and dinner. The others were given a placebo. After two months on the psyllium, LDL cholesterol fell 7.2 percent in the individuals following the low-fat diet and 6.4 percent in the individuals on the high-fat diet. The LDL cholesterol of the placebo-takers didn't change.

If you prefer to take psyllium in a breakfast cereal, you can select from Brand Buds or FiberWise. Bran Buds contain wheat bran, an insoluble fiber that promotes regularity and health of the colon, as well as soluble fiber.

Those who choose a psyllium supplement should follow the recommended dosage on the label. And, for maximum effect (as previously mentioned), they should take psyllium with meals. In a study at the University of Toronto, people with mildly high cholesterol who ate a psyllium-cereal for two weeks saw their cholesterol drop by 8 percent. But those who took psyllium powder, mixed with water, between meals had only a minor drop in cholesterol.

Caution: Too much psyllium can slow the absorption of certain kinds of heart and blood pressure medication. Also, if you've had an allergic reaction to laxatives--or if you have any kind of allergy at all--you should check with your doctor before taking psyllium. In rare cases, this fiber has caused anaphylaxis (a severe allergic reaction).

PECTIN: ANOTHER HEART-FRIENDLY FIBER

If you've heard of pectin, it's probably as an ingredient in jelly. But this gummy substance is found in most fruits and many vegetables, and nutritional scientists are discovering that it, too, can help reduce cholesterol level.

To recap, there are two kinds of fiber: soluble and insoluble. Soluble fiber has been proven to help lower blood cholesterol. Pectin, apparently accomplishes this by interfering with the body's absorption of cholesterol.

It may also affect certain enzymes in the liver that produce cholesterol.

Studies indicate that the more pectin you eat, the less cholesterol the liver produces.

In one two-month-long study, 27 people considered to be at moderate tohigh risk for coronary heart disease eat either 15 grams of pectin daily day (in capsule form) or a placebo. month. For the next month, the people switched--those consuming the pectin took the placebos, and vice versa.

Results: those who consumed the pectin supplements instead of the placebos lowered their total cholesterol an average of 7.6 percent--and bad LDL cholesterol dropped about 10.8 percent.

In another study, 14 miniature pigs were given a high-fat diet for more than a year--sufficient time for the little porkers to block their coronary arteries with plaque. For the subsequent nine months, half the pigs continued with this same fatty diet but were given plus 3 percent grapefruit pectin. The other half were fed the high-fat diet without added pectin.

At the end of the test, while the pectin had not appreciably lowered the animals' cholesterol levels, it had reduced the plaque buildup in the coronary arteries and aortas. The coronary arteries of the pigs who had taken no pectin had narrowed an average of 45 percent, while those of the pectin-fed pigs had narrowed only 24 percent. Another studied focused on the effects of grapefruit pectin on the cholesterol levels of 27 people--people deemed to be at moderate to high risk for coronary heart disease because of elevated cholesterol levels.

The men and women consumed either 15 grams (about three teaspoons) of grapefruit pectin in capsule form or a placebo every day for four weeks. Then for another four weeks, the people consuming the pectin took the placebo, and vice versa.

The results? Total cholesterol dropped an average of 7.6 percent, from 275 to 254 milligrams/deciliter, when they consumed the pectin supplement as opposed to the placebo. And their "bad" LDL cholesterol plummeted an average of 11 percent, from 195 to 174 milligrams/deciliter.

How much pectin is enough?

The therapeutic dose (enough to reduce blood cholesterol levels) for water-soluble fibers such as pectin is about 15 grams a day. So where can you get that much pectin into your diet?

* Fruits and vegetables. Veggies rich in pectin include carrots, lettuce, spinach, beets, brussels sprouts, cabbage, potatoes, onions and peas. Fruits include grapefruit, oranges, bananas, strawberries, peaches, apples, grapes and plums.

Grapefruit, whether red, white or pink, is one of the richest pectin sources, while also being loaded with vitamin C.

And go for the whole fruit or vegetable, not just the juice. The fiber of the fruit or vegetable contains more pectin than the juice. And you'll feel more satisfied after eating a whole fruit or veggie than after drinking a glass of juice.

MORE BENEFITS OF GRAPEFRUIT

Of course, some folks don't relish a grapefruit half every morning. But, with a little ingenuity, you can solve that problem.

Here are a few tips:

* Choose brightly colored grapefruit with thin, fine-textured skin.

Generally speaking, the thinner the skin, the juicier the grapefruit."

* Sprinkle a half grapefruit with brown sugar and bake it. This not only makes a tasty dessert, but tames the natural tartness.

* Serve grapefruit sections as an accompani-

ment to spicy foods such as chili.

* Drizzle a tablespoon of honey or maple syrup over slices of kiwi fruit and peeled sections of orange and grapefruit. Sprinkle the fruits with cinnamon and nutmeg, then serve over raw fresh spinach dressed lightly with olive oil.

* Use a "grapefruit supplement." ProFibe, a tasteless powder that contains grapefruit pectin and other water-soluble fibers, can be blended into beverages, sprinkled onto salads or cereals or mixed into baked goods.

Those with moderately elevated blood cholesterol might consume 15 grams of ProFibe daily. (To find out more about ProFibe, write to Cer-Burg Enterprises, P.O. Box 245, Hawthorne, FL 32640, or call 1-800-756-3999.)

A FIBER THAT BINDS FAT

Chitin is the most abundant natural fiber next to cellulose (to which it has certain similarities). The most abundant source of chitin is in the shells of shellfish such as crab and shrimp.

Research on the uses of chitin and chitosan flourished in the 1930s and early 1940s but the rise of synthetic fibers, like the rise of synthetic medicines, overshadowed the interest in natural products. Interest in natural products, including chitin and chitosan, gained a resurgence in the 1970s and has continued to expand ever since.

Like many other plant fibers, chitosan is not digestible; therefore it has no caloric value. No matter how much chitosan you ingest, its calorie count remains at zero--an obviously important property for any weight-loss product.

Unlike other plant fibers, however, chitosan's properties give it the ability to significantly bind fat, acting like a fat sponge in the digestive tract.

* Chitosan and Cholesterol

Chitosan has the capacity to lower LDL cholesterol while boosting HDL cholesterol. Laboratory tests performed on rats showed that chitosan depresses serum and liver cholesterol levels in cholesterol-fed rats without affecting performance. Japanese researchers have concluded that chitosan can effectively lower blood serum cholesterol levels with no apparent side effects.

A study reported in the American Journal of Clinical Nutrition found that chitosan is as effective in mammals as cholestryramine (a cholesterol-lowering drug) in controlling blood serum cholesterol without the deleterious side effects typical of cholestryramine.

In fact, chitosan effectively lowered cholesterol absorption more than guar gum or cellulose.

* How Chitosan Reduces LDL Cholesterol Levels.

Our bodies make bile acids in the liver using the cholesterol from LDL.

When chitosan binds bile acids, it increases the rate of LDL loss, thus improving the LDL to HDL ratio. If enough bile acids are bound, the fats are not solubilized, which prevents their digestion and absorption.

* Substances That Enhance the Action of Chitosan

1. Ascorbic Acid

Combining chitosan with ascorbic acid results in even less fat absorption and greater fecal fat losses. In one study the addition of ascorbic acid to a chitosan enriched diet increased fecal fat losses by 87 percent and decreased fat absorption by over 50 percent.

2. Citric Acid

In experiments with animals, adding citric acid to a chitosan-enriched diet resulted in a decreased feed consumption. The most likely explanation for this effect is that the citric acid may be enhancing the swelling action of chitosan, leading to a sense of fullness, producing satiety and appetite suppression.

3. Chelated Minerals

When fat is burned, heat and energy are released. If a lack of certain minerals exists, energy levels will drop. Minerals help to transport needed nutrients to depleted areas of the body, thereby stemming off the fatigue we so often experience after eating a fatty meal.

4. Essential Fatty Acids

Prostaglandins control and balance many body functions. The dietary building blocks for making Prostaglandins are the essential fatty acids (EFAs). EFAs reduce the synthesis of triglycerides and very low-density lipoproteins (bad cholesterol) in the liver. EFA supplementation coupled with a low-cholesterol, low-saturated fat in diet produces a complementary effect in lowering serum lipid levels.

* Is Chitosan Safe?

Chitosan has been used extensively in many industrial, health and food applications. Clinical studies have used amounts in the 3-6 grams per day range with no adverse effects. As with any fiber, a person is well advised to drink plenty of water. (Whenever taking any form of fiber, drinking at least 8 glasses of water per day is highly recommended.)

However, constipation or diarrhea may occur in some persons depending on their individual constitutions and on how well the Chitosan supplement was originally formulated.

And, because Chitosan can bind lipids and certain minerals, it is best to take essential fatty acid supplements, fat soluble vitamins and mineral supplements separate from Chitosan.

Other Cautions:

You should not take chitosan if you have any kind of shellfish allergy, are pregnant or are breast-feeding. And, if you are taking medication of any kind, check with your physician before taking chitosan, since some drugs maybe bound to the Chitosan.

* When to Take Chitosan:

The best way to take chitosan is before eating a high-fat meal.

EVEN IF YOU'RE NOT THIRSTY, DRINK!

You may need water, but not be thirsty.

How can this happen? Scientists have found that as a person grows older, especially a sedentary person, he or she may lose the sense of thirst. So if you're over 50 and don't exercise, your ability to sense the need to drink may decline even to the point where you become dehydrated.

Other bad things can happen. The body's water content can easily drop to the point where all perspiration stops. Cooling the skin by the evaporation of sweat is the body's natural response to being over-heated. If the body can't cool itself by perspiring, the core temperature can rise to a dangerous level.

At the same time, the kidneys can lack sufficient water to flush body waste out in urine.

How can you tell if you're dehydrated? One sign is that if your urine is brown or dark yellow and you aren't urinating at regular intervals, you may be suffering mild dehydration. This can especially be true if you are eating a high-fiber diet, which takes a large fluid intake for proper digestion.

Normally during the day the urine should be clear--and should be voided in significant amounts and reasonable intervals.

Luckily, though dehydration in older people can be quite dangerous, it can be easily prevented and even easily reversed. The first obvious solution is to drink water--eight glasses a day at a minimum (see below for broader recommendations). Other fluids may be okay. Herbal tea, carbonated water, orange juice and other fruit juices are good sources of water, but coffee and sodas with high caffeine act as a diuretic.

HOW MUCH WATER SHOULD YOU DRINK?

You may be astounded to learn Dr. Linus Pauling's prescription for water intake--more than three quarts daily! Which works out to a glass every hour.

At least a liter, he maintained, is necessary daily

to produce sufficient urine to carry off the harmful substances that have been extracted from the blood in the kidneys.

Another way to determine optimum water intake: Drink in ounces daily half your body weight in pounds. Example: If you weigh 180 pounds, you should take in ninety ounces of water daily, which, at 32 ounces per quart, works out to a little less than three quarts per day. Almost the same as Pauling's prescription.

A high water intake naturally leads to a high volume of urine. And this, Pauling says, reduces the burden on the kidneys, since it's easier to excrete a diluted urine than concentrated urine. Especially is this so for persons with kidney problems.

Also, with high water intake there is loss chance of forming crystals, or "stones," out of body fluids.

AVOID 'SOFT' WATER

There seems to be a link, however, between drinking soft water and coronary disease. Soft water has had its minerals removed, and certain minerals-- selenium and zinc, for instance--are required by the body for absorption of antioxidants, which are in turn necessary for keeping arteries disease-free.

It makes practical sense, therefore, not to drink either soft or distilled water, unless you're also taking a mineral supplement.

HOW FIBER MAKES OTHER FOODS OKAY

The exciting part is--brace yourself--fiber can improve your diet. Oat bran alone, or psyllium, or guar gum (or all three!) will help to make red meats and cheeses less damaging to the body.

With such bran eaten regularly with meals, there's no reason not to enjoy a good, rare steak when you want it. Indeed, make special note of this: the right "gel" makes virtually all other foods--except excess starch, overcooked foods and damaged fats--quite okay.

Sugars and starch, we have covered.

Overcooked food not only is devoid of enzymes, but when deeply discolored--"browned"--cannot be recognized by the body, and decays in the digestive tract.

Damaged fats may have been burned or are rancid from exposure to heat or air or both. These dangerous fats, present in pasteurized dairy, overcooked eggs and even in cosmetics, are time-bombs of free radical damage. You won't notice at first, but eventually, radical damage reveals itself to be the very process of aging. (See "Free Radicals and Heart Disease" in Chapter Four, if you missed it.)

BROWNED FOODS POSE RISK FOR DIABETICS

A 1996 study suggests browned foods in general also represent a particular hazard to diabetics.

These foods contain a high concentration of a toxic material called advanced glycated end products, or AGEs. AGEs produced naturally in the body are thought to be prime contributors to the deadly complications of diabetes, but no one had closely studied their role in the diet.

The AGEs in a meal containing browned foods are quickly absorbed by the body and can double or triple the concentration of AGEs in the bloodstream. The dietary chemicals are a particular risk for people who already have diabetic kidney damage, which prevents the body from clearing them rapidly.

The molecules of AGEs are formed when proteins in cells and the blood combine with sugars. This process occurs at a low rate in all people and may be part of the aging process, but it is accelerated in diabetics because of the high sugar levels in their bloodstreams. Diabetics typically have two to three times the normal level of AGEs in their blood.

AGEs are sticky, kind of like a molecular glue. They glom onto the insides of blood vessels, stiffening the arteries and leading to the formation of plaque and clots. In organs like the kidney, they clog up the tiny pores that normally remove wastes from the blood.

AGEs have also been known to occur in many cooked foods when sugars and protein are heated together. This browning process, known formally as the Maillard reaction, produces AGEs, but until this study they were not believed to be toxic, to be absorbed into the bloodstream or to have any biological effect other than imparting flavor and color.

IMPORTANCE OF GOOD DIGESTION

The free-radical problem appears to be one of digestion--and not faulty digestions only. Human beings the world around do not digest all of the proteins in complete-protein foods of animal source.

When these proteins are not perfectly broken down and assimilated, they remain in the intestines, where, in dark, warm moisture, they decay.

Always remember that good digestion is not a process of putrefaction.

Decaying meat is not digesting meat. Such deteriorating foods--some vegetable-source foods, too--then become toxic and cease to serve the body, poisoning it rather than feeding it.

It is extremely unfortunate and unnecessary that certain foods are so fanatically avoided when any food which is rather browned in cooking becomes unrecognizable to the digestive enzymes responsible for identification. And when any food, regardless of what it is or what its source, cannot be recognized enzymically, it is rejected. Enzymes determine what is known and what is unknown, and, therefore, what is used and not used by the body.

While over fifty-thousand different kinds of enzymes are necessary for human health, there is no one enzyme for recognizing every food in every body.

Thus overcooked vegetables are just as deadly to health, and perhaps far more so, than a seared steak.

The qualities of food and the care in their preparation are just as important to health as the kinds of food. Further, the balance of the diet can make or break the benefit from any kind of food.

FAST NUTRITIONAL REVIEW:

1. Rule out large amounts of carbohydrate (eat just a little more thanyour total protein);

2. Avoid sugar like the plague and heap on the sour things, as C and fresh lemons;

3. Do not eat damaged, burned or rancid fats.

4. Keep oils down to the essentials:

* Omegas-3, 6, and 9;

* Vitamins E, A and D;

* Small, or half-teaspoon amounts, of extra-virgin olive oil, well-protected flax-seed oil, cod-, shark- or salmon-liver oils, if well-protected from oxygen;

* Japanese rice-bran oil. Butter, especially raw butter, is excellent in small amounts.

* Viobin Wheat Germ Oil, which uniquely strengthens the T-factor of the heart and increases stamina.

FISHING FOR GOOD HEART HEALTH

Reports of low heart-disease death rates among populations who consume large amounts of fish have led to theories that the fat found in fish might reduce the risk of coronary artery disease.

In 1995, researchers from Seattle published a major study in which they obtained dietary histories of

334 patients who had experienced cardiac arrests. Analysis of food intake suggested that the cardiac-arrest victims ate less fish than the healthy control subjects. The researchers concluded that eating one fish meal a week reduced the risk of cardiac arrest by 50%. Eating two fish meals per month reduced the risk by 30%.

The researchers theorized that the type of fat provides the beneficial effects--and some fish offer more of this fat than others. For example, a typical serving of salmon--a fatty fish--has more than six times as much as leaner cod. Other fatty fish include herring, mackerel, and anchovies. Smaller amounts of the key fats are found in oysters, sardines, rainbow trout, albacore tuna and other seafood.

A natural heart-rhythm drug:

Several studies suggest that fish oil might be a natural heart-rhythm drug. Laboratory research indicates that fish oil might "stabilize" heart rhythms by influencing the flow of chemicals across the coverings of heart-muscle cells. This is especially encouraging since the drugs used to treat heart-rhythm abnormalities can have dangerous side effects.

FATTY FISH CUTS RISK OF HEART ATTACKS

New research indicates that lost one serving of fatty fish (such as salmon) per week can reduce the risk of cardiac arrest by as much as 70 percent.

A recent issue of The Journal of the American Medical Association featured a study from the University of Washington in Seattle that focused on the cardiac benefits of a polyunsaturated fatty acid found primarily in seafood. More than 300 individuals who had suffered primary cardiac arrest and nearly 500 population-based controls filled out food intake surveys.

Individuals in the two groups, who ranged in age from 24 to 74, were matched for age and sex.

Researchers found that individuals who ate the equivalent of 5.5 grams of Omega-3 fatty acids per month had an associated 50 percent reduction in the risk of primary cardiac arrest. Four 3-ounce servings of salmon contain approximately 5.96 grams of Omega-3 fatty acids, enough to reap the cardiac benefits.

Why the reduction in risk? Well, it seems that the Omega-3 fatty acids found in fatty fish are effective in increasing the levels of fatty acids in blood cell membranes. This, in turn, reduces the clumping of blood platelets and coronary spasm.

Even small increases in the percentage of Omega-3 fatty acids in the total fatty-acid level can substantially lower the risk of heart attack.

Researchers found that as the percentage of Omega-3 fatty acids increases, the risk of primary cardiac arrest decreases accordingly.

Researchers say that additional clinical trials to assess the effectiveness of increased fatty acid intake on cardiac arrest risk should take place in the near future.

FISH AND TRIGLYCERIDE CONTROL

Most experts agree that a high triglyceride level

is a warning sign in many patients who have a predisposition for coronary heart disease.

Fortunately, a high triglyceride level can usually be brought down with lifestyle changes. Some of the most common triglyceride-lowering strategies are losing weight, avoiding alcohol, refined carbohydrates and sugars and starting an exercise program.

But there's a new anti-triglyceride prescription available to physicians--fish.

Studies have shown that the cholesterol-lowering omega-3 fatty acids in fatty fish such as salmon and albacore tuna can help lower elevated triglycerides.

Some doctors recommend eating fish about twice a week. But you need to prepare the fish properly--broiled or steamed rather than fried.

Fish oil can also help lower triglycerides as well, according to William P. Castelli, M.D., medical director of the Framingham Cardiovascular Institute in Framingham, Mass. Research has showed that only fish oil can lower triglycerides to under 500 milligrams/deciliter in people whose triglycerides topped 1,000 milligrams/deciliter.

As little as three to four grams of fish oil a day may be all that's needed, Dr. Castelli concluded.

FOR BETTER OR WORSE: MARGARINE OR BUTTER?

Every attempt by science to "create" dairy products seems doomed to failure. By the turn of the century, scientists had chemically duplicated cows' milk. This "milk" was then fed to mice--which all died.

But when butter was found guilty of containing cholesterol--and it was a hard fat, to boot--so here came margarine to take its place. Now any fool can churn milk and make butter, it is not a laboratory feat of accomplishment. But margarine was a scientific miracle.

The only problem, as we see further down that road, is that the body doesn't know what it is.

People who don't have the enzymes for "recognizing" dairy products don't know what butter is either. But that isn't everyone.

However, it seems now that we don't have the recognition factors in us to handle margarine and never did have.

It used to be thought that butter had a slightly higher incidence of heart disease associated with its consumption, while margarine showed higher cancer. But, as you'll see from the Framingham Heart Study results detailed in the next section, even that pro-margarine myth has dissolved under laboratory scrutiny. Butter wins again.

And, of course, it tastes better, too. Always did. But again we must emphasize: if you are not a cholesterol sensitive, eat the butter, and not to worry. If you are a "sensitive," increase fiber and niacin--and enjoy the butter along with your toast and eggs.

It should be obvious that with large differences in how individuals handle food, it would be ridiculous to channel and harass an entire nation and an entire culture into avoiding certain taboo foods in the delusion that this will earn millions of people absolution from all disease, fat and premature death.

NO RISK WITH BUTTER?

There were surprising results from a study of 865 men participating in the long-running Framingham Heart Study conducted by Harvard Medical School study. Men who ate five teaspoons of margarine a day had twice the heart disease risk of men who didn't eat margarine.

The study looked at butter and found no increased risk.

Despite this evidence (of course!), many doctors continue to recommend staying away from butter, or to recommend lower-fat margarines--or olive oil, which has monounsaturated fats.

What would you expect?

CHOLESTEROL-KILLING MARGARINE?

There may, however, be something good to say about margarine. The London Times reported on a Finnish-produced margarine that claims to reduce blood cholesterol levels. This product costs several times the price of normal margarine and will not be available for export until 1997.

The margarine Benecol was publicized in a report in the New England Journal of Medicine in November, 1995, where researchers concluded that daily consumption of 25 grams--the amount spread on two slices of toast--reduced total cholesterol in the bloodstream by 10 percent and the level of the more harmful LDL cholesterol by 14 percent. (This could be enough to reduce the likelihood of a heart attack by a third, according to the report.) The higher the cholesterol levels before consumption of Benecol began, the greater was the reduction.

The Finnish manufacturer, Raisio, has not been able to keep up with local demand. Its share price quickly doubled and international investors have been piling in since the product was spotlighted by an international securities analyst.

In fact, an extra processing unit was built to increase production of plant sterols on which Benecol, a "full-fat margarine", depends.

The manufacturers point out that Benecol is itself a fat and should therefore be used to replace, and not supplement, other dietary fat.

The new spread's inventor, Ingmar Wester, spent seven years working to introduce plant sterols-- which block cholesterol absorption--into mass food production. "Margarine is just one possible way of administering plant sterols," he has stated. "We are also now looking at chocolate bars, ice cream and mayonnaise."

EVEN 'GOOD' OILS CAN GO 'BAD'

It's important to keep oils, whether liquid or capsule, cold and airless. All oils, whether in liquid or capsule form, must be kept sealed and cold at all times, until eaten.

Oxygen damages oils, making them rancid, causes free radicals and makes them dangerous to health. Oxygen, even in a few days, can penetrate capsules and form the free radicals which age the body. Capsules are excellent for carrying to work and taking at lunchtime. But we're talking a convenience of hours, here; not days.

Exposed oils can become rancid in so little time it's frightening.

Leftovers, even when chilled, are almost always rancid; though precautions to exclude heat and air may make leftovers practical and safe. Leave no oil-containing foods exposed to air--for your heart's sake.

Remember: dish-covers do not exclude air!

RED MEAT RECONSIDERED

One of the bad things about red meat is that it does not, and apparently cannot, perfectly digest in the lower intestines. Or it is not digested perfectly upon arrival, and nothing in the intestines can cope with that--except:

* Soluble brans and vitamin B-6.

Vitamin B-6 is a mild form of hydrochloride and aids in digesting difficult proteins.

Without these foods, a steak will rot in the intestines. When this happens, the system is over-loaded with toxins that seep through the intestinal walls, enter the bloodstream and are carried to the liver to be taken care of. (Constipation, unfortunately, guarantees that every bit of the toxin gets carried off to the wrong place.)

There is no way that blood can oppose these infusions. Toxins are toxins, and they are sent to the liver. Spoiled foods, stemming from the lower intestines, can thus actually reach up and enter the liver.

The effect of these toxins on the liver can be disastrous--the liver may cease entirely its production of that heart-protector, lecithin. Lecithin dissolves fats and is one of our major bulwarks against excess fats of all kinds in the diet. Lecithin is a solvent. Though itself an oil, it breaks up plaque in the arteries, helps to lower both pressure and cholesterol, as well as comprising two-thirds of the dry weight of the brain.

Thus with lecithin-production knocked out by toxins, the body, brain and heart are directly and adversely affected.

This is the pathway whereby red meat has received its bad name, and whereby it is said to cause heart trouble and even contribute to senility. The fat in beef is not the direct cause of the difficulty, for, were the liver not damaged primarily by toxins from the intestines, beef fat would be no problem.

After a lifetime of abuse, the liver cannot put these toxins "out of their misery" and shuts down other functions instead--among them, its genius for making lecithin.

LECITHIN--LIFE-AND HEART-SAVER

We must have lecithin, just as we must have cholesterol. How do we know we must have this interesting food? Because a healthy liver makes it. (Though most livers make too little lecithin or make none at all.)

The connection between the two--lecithin and cholesterol--is interesting. Both are forms of fat. But lecithin is water-dispersible. It has the capacity to saponify (turn into soap) cholesterol and other fats.

Because plaque is primarily a collapsed blob of cholesterol, lecithin in the bloodstream literally scrubs it away. Lecithin breaks up plaque.

PLAQUE ATTACK REVISITE

Plaque is a substance that accumulates within the lumen of arteries. (The lumen is the open part of blood vessels.) When the lumen becomes clogged (as we've mentioned several times), blood flow is cut and tissues begin to starve for all the nutrients of life. This is one of the sad beginnings of heart disease.

So it is critically important to keep your lumen fully open and clear. For that is the very space through which your blood flows.

When low-density lipoproteins (LDL's, the bad kind) splash against arterial walls, they don't rebound, like high-density lipoproteins (HDLs).

They smear along the sides. This thick substance collects calcium and debris of any kind drifting along in the blood current.

Such heaps of plaque can merge with other plaque. More can begin to build upon the opposite wall in the same area and, finally, encircle the lumen itself. Your blood then flows through a tube which is getting narrower and narrower as its walls get thicker and thicker. Like any garden hose, the pressure within has to go up.

This whole tragic story, a process of degeneration, takes its toll against the heart.

All too often this coating of plaque in the artery leaves little opening through which blood can surge and other injuries ensue. Total occlusion may cause a number of complications and even a fatal disaster.

LECITHIN BEATS THE 'WONDER DRUGS'

Surely, any natural substance which dissolves these deadly plaques must be valued highly. Lecithin is such a substance. It is found also in plants, particularly in soy beans, and the extracted lecithin can be purchased, added to foods and used successfully to fight excessive cholesterol.

Being a kind of oil, lecithin is subject to rancidity when exposed to air and must be protected like any other food oil.

When people lack lecithin--that is, when the liver has ceased to make it--the diet should be richly supplemented with this cholesterol-fighter.

In trials with drugs purported to lower high blood pressure or to remove plaque, lecithin always comes out ahead, does the job best. Lecithin does it faster, safer (with fewer deaths) and fewer side effects (in fact, none) than any known drug.

Naturally, once this became known (over forty years ago), further tests on drugs tended to exclude lecithin. Why let someone play who always wins?

WHERE TO GET YOUR LECITHIN

You can eat lecithin in granules; or as a thick syrup; or in capsule or chewable wafer form. While it is a tremendous assist to the arteries and the health of the heart, taking it this way does not entirely replace the economy to the body of making its own. Bear in mind that correcting your dietary lecithin does not necessarily correct other infractions which shut off lecithin-production in the liver in the first place.

Which brings us back to red meats and their bad reputation. Toxins in the liver caused by putrefying foods cause the liver to shut down lecithin production. Eliminating red meats doesn't invariably restore liver function and avoiding such meats may be just one more nutritional loss.

(See "Good Things About Red Meat" farther on.)

Ideally, lecithin production in the liver should, if possible, be restored. In any case, supplementing your diet with edible lecithin is prudent housekeeping for plaque already in the arteries and a sound preventative against future plaque.

TAKING SOY TO HEART

We mentioned that a prime source of lecithin is soy beans. This is one reason that many experts say soy's ability to clear cholesterol from the circulation is unsurpassed by any other foodstuff.

Soy protein is a part of the humble bean that, at least in the U.S., is more often fed to animals than humans.

Good dietary sources of this protein are tofu (soy bean curd), soy flour and other dry and moist preparations. (Soy sauce contains only a trace and has the drawback of being loaded with sodium.)

Researchers from the University of Kentucky at Lexington found that those who ate an average of 47 grams daily had a 12.9% fall in harmful low-density lipoprotein (LDL) and a 9.3% drop in total cholesterol. (Their HDL-cholesterol stayed about the same.)

Italy has specialized in soy protein science. In fact, Italian cardiologists have long prescribed soy protein to both children and adults with some inherited forms of hypercholesterolemia (elevated cholesterol). The Italian National Health Service even provides it free to some families.

How does soy protein work?

Evidence suggests that soy boosts the activity of LDL receptors, which snatch bad cholesterol and deliver it to the liver where it is broken down for excretion. (In addition, soy is high in folate, protein, omega-3 fatty acids and minerals.)

Although studies showed positive results for people who ate 47 grams of soy protein daily, some experts believe that 20 to 25 grams (or 5 to 6 ounces of firm tofu) may be enough to lower cholesterol levels. In addition, tofu is rich in iron and magnesium and is an excellent source of vegetable protein.

Some tofu even comes fortified with calcium.

The large amounts of soy protein in Asian diets indicates that this food is safe, but many Americans do not like the "beany" aftertaste of many soy foods. Plain tofu is definitely an acquired taste--and may even seem tasteless. This is the white, custard-like (but not custard-tasting) food madefrom curdled soy milk which is, in turn, made from cooked soybeans. The resulting curds are drained and pressed into cakes, much like cheese is.

Fortunately, the food industry has recently been successful in developing soy proteins that are bland enough to be unnoticeable by many consumers.

While tofu can be sliced, diced or mashed and then added to soups, stir-fries, casseroles and sandwiches, it can also be used as the main ingredient to build a dish around.

Here is a tofu recipe that's easy to get down:

HAWAIIAN SMOOTHIE

1 cup pineapple juice, unsweetened

1 cup crushed pineapple (fresh or use one 8-ounce   can)

2 tablespoons apricot jam

One 10.5-ounce package lite silken tofu, firm

1 ripe banana

Combine all ingredients in a blender. Whip until smooth. Chill or blend in a few ice cubes. Serve cold. Makes two (10-ounce) servings.

If you just can't abide tofu, however, you also get your protein via soy milk or add soy flour to baked goods, and soy protein can be added to ravioli, lasagna and other dishes (how the Italians eat it).

Estimated Amounts of Soy

Product	Soy Protein
8 oz soy milk	4 to 10 grams
4 oz of tofu	8 to 13 grams
1 oz soy flour	10 to 13 grams
1 oz isolated soy protein	23 grams
1/2 cup textured soy protein	11 grams
3.2 oz of meat analogue	18 grams

GOOD THINGS ABOUT RED MEAT

As a general basis for diet, avoid any one food in excess. While red meats are high in fat, they do provide ten times the vitamin B-12 found in poultry and fish. This elusive vitamin (at root a bacterium that we are supposed to "catch") is our prime anti-anemia factor and a brain-memory factor, too.

Dark meats have, around the world, seemed to provide more strength than white meats, possibly because of the B-12, but certainly because of the presence in red meats of red cells which, if the meat is not overcooked by heat, are readily absorbed by the body and well used.

Red meats, cooked rare, are known for their power in building new blood. If not much fat is taken, red meat is a superior blood-builder.

Further, red meats, especially tough cuts, if not heat-damaged, provide cartilaginous matter which is necessary for strong tendons and muscles (this does include the heart, which is solid muscle) and which is almost entirely missing from the modern, semi-vegetarian diet.

And the red cells in a rare steak directly feed your own bloodstream with essentials, including iron and all the elements necessary for your making more blood.

Of course, beef is an excellent source of high-quality protein and a good source of heme iron (the kind most usable by the body). For years (before the big scare) physicians actually prescribed red meat, rare steaks and such, for pregnant mothers needing to strengthen their blood.

There can be no doubt about it: Red meats in moderation are an extremely potent (and enjoyable) food for most people.

B-6 TO THE RESCUE

Vitamin B-6 is a major "heart food." How? This vitamin (as we said before) is a mild form of hydrochloric acid and has the characteristic of being able to digest the very proteins which give human beings so much trouble. As an HCL, B-6 can begin its work upon proteins in the stomach and almost everywhere else along the line. Some nutritionists believe that it should be against the law to eat a steak without at least 300 milligrams of B-6 beside the plate.

ALL-BEEF DIETS

There have been many studies of Eskimos and Arctic explorers who lived for long periods on only meat and suffered no dietary deficiencies. One study focussed on two explorers who, for one year, ate nothing but meat (beef, lamb, veal, pork, chicken, liver, kidney, brain, bacon and bone marrow). The study concluded that the two were in as good health at the end of the year as at the beginning.

ANTI-BEEF PREJUDICE

Nutritionists daily see vegetarians who desperately need a blood-rare steak, but they hesitate to suggest it, because the prejudice against eating beef often makes the social aspect of the encounter uncomfortable. The assumed virtue on this point sometimes approaches religious fervor.

Such prejudices can and do lead to serious nutritional losses, and the loss of meat cartilage can be cited as just one of them.

Why some folks are afraid of the cow:

Understandably, some people fear that any kind of drug which may have been shot into a steer is still right in the meat. And yet, even when assured that the animal has come from a far land, South America or Australia, say, which use neither steroids nor crop sprays, the prejudice has so darkened the cow's name that red meat is avoided.

We have actually seen a man who spent ten years as a drunk, smoked for two decades and who has suffered brain-damage from drugs and tars, suppose that a cow which has eaten only grass and rainwater and stood under the sky for six years is more poisoned than himself. This verges on the incomprehensible.

Further, dark meats have been observed over many centuries to invest greater strength into the body than is gained from white. The source of this strength is believed to be in the pigment itself.

In any case, beef appears to have two disastrous faults, bearing on human diet: We can't completely digest the proteins, and it is rich in cholesterol-bearing fats.

IN DEFENSE OF FAT AND CHOLESTEROL

Another word on fats is therefore justified. During the days of sailing ships, it was well understood by sailors that the strength from meat was in the fat, not the muscle tissue. Men aboard ship fought for

the fatty parts because of the very true (and now scientifically proven) fact that fat is about forty times
more efficient as energy than carbohydrate.

Men have fought for the fatty parts of meat and
have killed for them. If fat is energy, then why, we must
wonder, are overweight people so frequently dead
tired all the time? They would seem to have tons of
fuel. Why won't the body burn it? A perfect storehouse
of energy, yet no energy at all.

As said before, while indulging excessive starch,
the body will not turn to the fat, because one's fat is,
after all, one's own tissue. But that fat is elsewhere,
behind lock and key, while the glycogen, sugar in solid
form, is right there in the liver. And even that will not
be available if high starch keeps insulin elevated too
frequently.

Those sailors did not gorge on starch, there was-
n't that much of it. And there wasn't time to sit around
munching. Nobody on board could be a "couch potato."

Thus, these sailors' bodies were lean. They
quickly ran through their stores of glycogen--if any
was stored--and under the labors of sailing a vessel
on the high seas, their metabolisms resorted to their
own fat for vigor, keeping such seamen notoriously
strong, lean and unbelievably energetic.

At least that's the romantic lore. So let's look at
this from a more modern point of view:

To digest any oil, any fat, requires bile. To make
bile, to digest fat, your liver must produce something-
-and guess what that is:

Cholesterol!

Not only does every cell of your body contain its

small portion of cholesterol as a necessity of life, your liver must make more, to make bile, to digest oil. You must digest oil, because only digested oil absorbs liquid calcium. And only when liquid calcium is absorbed by digested oil can this now-whitish oil, carrying its store of calcium, enter the lacteals of the small intestines, rise through the spinal section of your immune system, reach your vena cava and pour directly into your heart--where these essentials must go if you are to go on living.

If you starve your body for cholesterol, it might just decide upon its own to make more. Further, as we've seen, the avoidance diet notoriously fails to lower cholesterol.

The problem then is not that cholesterol, even bad cholesterol, is bad--it's absolutely necessary for life; avoiding it doesn't work. You might as well eat what you want and accept the fact that collecting it and getting rid of its excess by eating the fiber found in common foods is, after all, nature's best and only system for dealing with this endless, ongoing problem.

But suppose you continue avoiding cholesterol and living in fear of it?

If your liver does not step up production of cholesterol, how are you going t digest oil? Without bile (a common problem) how will you digest vitamins A and D and E? How will you survive without metabolizing the essential oils, omega-3, 6 and 9?

It should be clear that a more livable, reasonable, rational and comfortable day-to-day system must be found than living in fear, dread and revulsion of food.

WE'RE NOT SELLING BEEF HERE

The purpose of this section on soluble brans is not to promote red meats or animal gluttony; but is to relieve the pressure born of unnecessary deprivation. And also peer-group scorn, when people feel shamed into giving up perfectly good foods. Yes, meat is a good food--if you know how to prepare it, eat it, how much to eat, and how to protect yourself in reasonable ways from known disadvantages.

Buyer's Guide to Lean Beef: If you're going to start eating red meat again, or just want to adjust your intake to fit a lower-fat, low-cholesterol diet, here are three shopping and serving suggestions:

1. Pick the leanest cuts. For pork, make it tenderloin, leg or shoulder.

For lamb, choose the arm and loin. The leanest beef cuts are usually stamped "USDA select." "Select" on average contains 20 percent less fat than "choice" and 40 percent less than "prime." Extra-lean ground beef contains just 10 percent fat based on weight.

2. Visually estimate the fat content of any cut of meat by checking out the white marbling. Marbling equals fat.

3. Trim visible fat before cooking.

THE LEANEST CUTS

The following beef cuts of beef are usually the leanest (calculated for three ounces cooked):

MEAT	FAT (G.)	CALORIES
Eye of round	4.2	143
Top roast	4.2	153
Tip round	5.9	157
Top sirloin	6.1	165
Chuck roast	7.6	189
Top loin	8	176
Flank	8.6	176
Tenderloin	8.6	177

And, if you're really interested, you can find domestic beef raised without the use of hormones, at around 7% fat content, leaner than even extra lean ground beef found in most supermarkets. One Texas ranch, B3R Brand Beef, distributes to many health-food and specialty stores. For information on the distributor nearest you, call B3R at (817) 937-3668.)

The quotient of what it costs you in terms of what you get from beef can be decidedly in your favor--as it should have been all along, and was until modern times, when heart disease mounted to epidemic proportions.

There's more to be said on how to use brans and other nutrients, and even timing, to get the best from the foods you eat, as our next chapter will disclose.

Our objective? Better health, a stronger, more durable heart and a longer, more enjoyable life--that's all.

X. FOOD SUPPLEMENT FUNDAMENTALS

NUTRITION: SIMPLICITY VS. COMPLEXITY

Conclusions must be drawn on the matter of simplicity versus complexity.

Heavily boiled lime (or lemon) juice does not prevent death by scurvy.

Fresh juice does.

White rice does not prevent death from beriberi. Brown, whole rice does.

Strained or frozen, reconstituted orange juice does not lower cholesterol and help fight heart disease. Fresh orange juice--with pulp present--does.

Natural beers, as found largely in Europe, contain important B-complexvitamins. Big American brewers remove the B-vitamins essential for health. Indeed, without the natural yeast-fed vitamins in the beverage, there is less justification for beer in the diet.

Even so, researchers have found five or six ounces of beer near bedtime improve the sleep--and hence heart rest--of oldsters. (And any alcoholic beverage, in such quantity, has a certain benefit on hearth health--see "Alcohol and Your Heart" in Chapter 13.) A big mug of brew (over five or six ounces), however, is too much. If this were vitamin-rich beer instead of the devitalized, it could in this usage be classed virtually as a health food.

But notice, both common sense and complexity are at work in such a solution.

Whole, raw milk is better for you, butterfat and all, than is low-fat pasteurized milk, for the same reasons--though these classic instances are but the briefest examination of the mountains of research into every area of food, nutrition and health which await your discovery.

VALUE OF READING

It would not be untrue to list the reading of health-food and nutritional literature, reports and research papers as a health food in its own right. Read! We hope our book will only whet your appetite. Find out for yourself, rather than settling for someone else's word on matters of heart health (even ours). It has been our observation after working with hundreds of heart patients that those prosper most who boldly take charge of their own cases.

Of these many hundreds, those fare worst who consign their health, heart and their very lives into the hands of a physician. When these people convert to the more sane, workable approach, they tell us the same thing: "I didn't begin to get better until I took charge of my own health. I've made myself well."

DAILY FOOD SUPPLEMENTATION SHOULD BE COMPLEX

In fact, as complex as you can make it. Because our bodies are infinitely complex, every reasonable measure should be taken to supply them with all essentials.

There is a single hitch, however: Nobody can actually claim that all needs are finally and completely known, defined and isolated.

In diet, as well as in life overall, we are always dealing with the unknowns; and if you think about it, difficulties are ultimately what life is all about. There is a tremendous challenge in meeting each issue. Further, as in human culture, without the problems, there could be no romance, no charm, no zest. Thus, without spinning off into confusion in response to complexities and problems, we can relax and enjoy, because there are simple remedies, solutions which rack focus into clear-cut lines.

NUTRITIONALLY COMPLEX FOODS ARE EASY-TO-PREPARE

We must have real food that has lived, and hopefully is still alive, at least enzymically. Isn't this obvious by now?

Why sit down to a table loaded with nothing but cooked, baked and boiled foods? It's so much easier to place all sorts of fresh, raw foods out for a meal, and it's tastier, more satisfying. We don't need three kinds of bread.

For instance, a half of a not-too-done baked potato serves and balances best with a rational serving of meat or fowl or fish that has not been cremated or buried in a rich, fatty sauce.

Let raw fruits and vegetables predominate, with cells and nutrients not destroyed, all enzymes still active. The simplest raw food is in itself complete--and at its most complex.

The instant you start peeling away too much, crushing and thinning, sieving and refining, you are making your food more dainty, pretty--and deadly. You are simplifying, when it started out, before it was damaged, as complex as nature could make it.

SERVING FOOD FOR MAXIMUM NUTRITION

Even with baked sweet potatoes, which are delicious and loaded with nutrients (including soluble fiber, by the way, good for the heart), why not shave off thin slices of the sweet potato raw, or grate some onto your salad, so you get the full, complex chemistry?

When serving corn on the cob, make it golden corn when possible. Before cooking, shave and scrape off some and eat it raw as a small side-dish. Raw golden corn is one of our prime sources of that heart medicine, Co-enzyme Q-10. (More about this later.)

This isn't just a "raw craze." It's a primary, earthy recontact with that world of nature from which all live things spring. Your food is at its most complex before it is damaged by paring, heat and refining.

The marvel of this is that these foods, found right in our kitchens, have been of supreme benefit for lo, these many years. Most of us have never known that we held the very remedies right there in our hands, our refrigerators, our shopping bags, all this time. Naive and unknowing, we have most often put these benefits to death before they had the chance to enter our bodies, and join our bloodstreams, creating strength and health.

Simply placing the raw forms of these usually cooked foods on the table is the simplest nurturing of the heart known. Eat these good foods for their delicious and complex benefit--then go ahead and cook the portions you like, and eat those for other pleasures and qualities.

EVEN RAW FOODS LACK NUTRIENTS

We can, and should, eat food as fresh as raw as we palatably can. But, despite what certain anti-nutritionists keep repeating, we still need supplementation.

Because of ten-million stresses, because we live in a modern world unlike anything known over the last fifty-thousand years, it is essential to try for increased support in the known areas.

We do know that vitamin A, and B and C, and so on, replace nutrients lost in food handling, delays, poor refrigeration and even in soil losses. We need not list the sixty known causes of nutritional loss in foods which appear to be in perfect condition. We have already discussed the deliberate de-vitaminizing of cattle fodder to produce low-vitamin butter.

We forgot to mention, however, that commercial fertilizers invariably are inferior to the purely natural by-products of healthy cattle.

But when cattle are fed a poor diet, the manure they produce is less useful on soil, and such soil then produces inferior food crops. Such badly fed animals upon poor soil do not offer a fair or honest or accurate comparison with commercial additives.

It is even claimed that ocean toxins, a modern difficulty in all sea foods, affect algae, an almost perfect food. Some careful customers are turning to algae produced only in freshwater lakes in order to avoid food-chain contaminants.

No single fault, however, is quite as germane here in this discussion as our basic, overall need to supplement even an excellent diet with known, tested food supplements.

CURE BY FOOD ALONE

An anecdote may help to make our point:

A psychiatrist glanced into his waiting room and quickly withdrew. He had a problem. He had been overscheduled. There were dozens of patients sitting there, needing immediate psychiatric help. There was no time for extensive interviews covering weeks, months of time.

It was almost a joke. Here he was, the psychiatrists, while out there were the patients, coming to him for help. And he couldn't cope!

He had to do something, and fast.

This particular shrink (an unusual chap, you will see) decided that somehow, by some means, he would do something for everyone.

He ordered a catered lunch. He stipulated the health foods he wanted, abalanced diet, no trash foods. He also devised megadoses of all the known vitamins and minerals.

Presenting an entire waiting-room of patients, many of them in dire need of stability, rationality, reassurance, counseling and other psychiatric care, with a meal, plus strong food supplements, might appear foolish, if not a downright cop-out.

But everybody took the food and swallowed the supplements--like medication, as a matter of course.

Then he rescheduled them for individual appointments.

At least, he thought, he'd done something. Nobody had to sit there in a blind stupor. And certainly nobody would get worse until he could see them one at a time.

Oddly, when everybody showed up for their appointments, they were somehow a little better, their conditions improved.

Meal by meal, this continued. Eventually, in about six weeks, most of the patients were in fine shape. A high percent needed no further care, except a good nutritional program and the others on an out-patient basis.

The psychiatrists stated that while many disorders simply disappeared, the benefit was solid. "Helping these people was more important than knowing what was wrong with them," he concluded. Perhaps he, himself, was suffering from something akin to a "diagnosis disease." Once he got over that, he was able to help his patients dramatically and quickly.

This did not obviate further, even prolonged, psychiatric counseling and therapy for some. But the bottom line, once again, was that good food and megadoses of food supplements cured a high percentage of what appeared to be psychiatric problems.

Again, the meals emphasized complexity. Not food by itself, but with complex supplementation. And not with supplements alone, but complex food.

And guess what? You don't have to be a mental patient to set forth upon such a program.

DIAGNOSIS SECONDARY TO HEALING

As in our little anecdote about the clinic, diagnosis drops considerably in importance when immediate healing is urgent.

In that case, we dismiss exact knowledge of just why and how your cholesterol is high, or why you catch cold every winter.

To put it bluntly, who cares?

Lower the cholesterol and become immune to colds. There are ways to achieve such goals, and some we have discussed.

ABCs OF VITAMINS AND MINERALS

For much of the 20th century, it was thought that most Americans derived all the vitamins and minerals they needed from the foods they consumed. Recent evidence, however, clearly point to the need for in additional vitamins and minerals. There are three reasons for this:

1.The average American diet is packed with

calorie-rich but nutritionally insubstantial food. We simply do not eat enough whole grains, fruits and vegetables to obtain even the minimum amounts of some of the essential vitamins and minerals.

2. Our modern lifestyles and environment use up nutrients in quantities beyond what even the healthiest diet may replace. Example: pollutants deplete the body of antioxidants, stress lowers our supply of vitamins B and C, food dyes and preservatives block vitamin B-6 and folate, and heavy metals in the soil, sea may interfere with our trace mineral nutrition.

3. The conventional standard of vitamin and mineral requirements, set by the Food and Nutrition Board of the National Research Council, is vastly understated. These U.S. Recommended Daily Allowances (RDA) have undergone several revisions since first established in the 1940s, and are undergoing another update in the wake of overwhelming evidence suggesting that larger amounts of certain vitamins--principally antioxidants--can help prevent many diseases, including cancer and heart disease.

How vitamins and minerals work to maintain body functions:

Vitamins are organic substances found in plants and animals. Generally speaking, the body can't manufacture vitamins, so we must obtain them through the diet or through supplementation. There are approximately 14 vitamins considered vital to life, and several other nutrients whose roles are being studied.

Each vitamin carries out specific functions, and the lack of a certain vitamin can lead to subtle biochemical problems. Example: low vitamin D intake can lead to problems in calcium metabolism such as osteoporosis and, in its severe childhood form, can lead to the degenerative bone condition called rickets. Some vitamins, such as E and B-6, affect all cells and functions in the body without having a specific deficiency disease associated with them.

Minerals, meanwhile, are inorganic substances found in the earth's crust.

Carried into the soil and ground-water, they are taken up by plants and consumed by humans. Of the more than 60 different minerals found in the body, 22 are considered essential. Seven--including calcium, chloride, magnesium, phosphorus, potassium, sodium and sulfur--are considered major minerals.

Others, called trace minerals, are found in tiny amounts in the body, but they are nonetheless important.

Several nutritive substances are especially important to cardiovascular health. These include the antioxidants (vitamins C, E and beta-carotene and minerals zinc and selenium), vitamin B-6, niacin, sodium, potassium and magnesium.

Special note on magnesium: This mineral lowers LDL and raises HDL, tones down the sympathetic nervous system, in a manner similar to the cardiac drugs called beta-blockers, and slows down the processes that lead to atherosclerosis, platelet aggregation, and fibrin clotting in the arterial wall. Finally, magnesium frequently helps vitamin B-6 carry out its all-important functions.

Multiple studies have linked low magnesium levels with atherosclerosis, heart attacks, high blood pressure, arrhythmias, and even mitral valve prolapse syndrome. There is even data suggesting that prenatal magnesium deficiency is responsible for infant deaths due to cardiovascular causes.

Magnesium is found in complex carbohydrates, especially wheat bran, raw leafy green vegetables, nuts and bananas. There is even convincing evidence that magnesium is as important as calcium in the prevention of osteoporosis.

REVAMPING RDAs

Almost everyone agrees that it's time to revamp the RDAs--the

FDA's list of Recommended Daily Allowances of vitamins and minerals. That minutiae-filled table of numbers and nutrients was first drawn up almost 60 years ago by the government folks who set nutrition policy in the United States.

RDAs were established in 1941 at the request of the War Department.

Military leaders wanted to know what to put in rations and how to beef up the many malnourished enlistees.

Revising the list is normally done about every five to 10 years, and was last done in 1989. However, there is no money to fund the project and no consensus about how to do it should the money suddenly appear.

But with the great advances in nutritional research, obviously that list is seriously out of date.

But for the last 20 years, more and more research has been devoted to the effects of nutrients on developing chronic diseases, such as cardiovascular disease. And many nutrition experts are eager to see a new set of RDAs that would have more impact on reducing the chronic diseases that kill so many

Americans.

Some of the controversy surrounding vitamin levels includes:

Vitamin E: Several studies show that taking daily doses more than seven times the current RDA results in a 40% decreased risk of heart disease.

Vitamin C: Studies show that 380 milligrams (six times the current RDA) could help reduce breast cancer by as much as 16%. Doses of 250 to 500 milligrams might also help reduce the risk of several other cancers.

Folic acid: According to the U.S. Department of Health and Human Services, more than doubling the RDA for women in their reproductive years could help reduce neural tube birth defects by at least half.

VITAMIN BUYER'S GUIDE

When you walk into a health-food store, or the vitamin section of a pharmacy, without taking a single pill you can be overdosed by the volume and variety of all those bottles on all those shelves. What should you buy, how much, which brand and size? Here's a start at clearing away confusion:

All makers of vitamins and minerals use the same raw materials. The real difference between brands is what additional ingredients are used--for instance, sugar, preservatives or coloring--and what ingredients are used for the tablet or capsule.

Example: some gelatin capsules are derived from vegetable sources, while others (the majority) use animal sources.

The majority of vitamin C sold is derived from corn and rice.

Vitamins, minerals and other supplements in tablet form are manufactured.

A supplement may contain only one vitamin or mineral, like vitamin C or chelated zinc, or may be a combination of vitamins and minerals, such as a multiple mineral or multi-vitamin. The manufacturer mixes the appropriate blend of raw materials and shapes it into tablets, capsules or other forms.

Another common question vitamin shoppers confront is: How long does it take a pill to dissolve after it's swallowed? There is no simple answer to that, however. It depends on the individual metabolism.

For example, age, illness, physical condition or activity level can contribute to assimilation of a supplement. Manufacturers do subject their products to what they call "disintegration tests," attempting to duplicate the action of the digestive tract.

GLOSSARY OF VITAMIN LABELS

In reading labels at a health food store, you may find yourself dizzied and bewildered by unfamiliar terms. So here is a brief rundown of some of the puzzling lingo:

BINDERS--Substances that give cohesive qualities to powdered materials.

They hold the ingredients together for tablet formulation. Some common binders are cellulose, a food grade binder; and providone or plasdone, inert granulating agents.

CHELATION--The process by which minerals are bonded to an amino acid. The body absorbs amino acids more easily than minerals, so this process enhances the absorption of minerals.

DISINTEGRANTS--These are added to the formulation to help the tablet disintegrate after consumption, thereby releasing the active ingredients.

Common disintegrants include several modified cellulose derivatives, which work by swelling when wet.

EXCIPIENTS--Various inert substances added to give the desired consistency or form for tableting. Vitamin tablets cannot be manufactured without excipients. Some common excipients are: binders, fillers, lubricants and disintegrants.

FILLERS--Inert materials added to the tablets to increase their bulk, in order to make them fit a particular size tablet mold for compression. Some common fillers are calcium phosphate and cellulose.

IU's--International Units, commonly used as a measurement of vitamins A and E and beta-carotene. International Units are an expression of potency while milligrams are a measurement of weight. 25,000 IU's of beta-carotene are equivalent to 15 mg.

LUBRICANTS--Inert material added in every small amounts (usually less than 1%) to the powder blend to prevent the compressed tablet from sticking to the tablet punches and dies. Common lubricants include vegetable stearin (similar to vegetable shortening) and magnesium stearate.

SYNERGISTIC--From the Greek word "synergia," meaning "joint work."

Substances are synergistic when they work

together as a team to produce an effect greater than the sum of their individual effects, i.e., vitamin C, rosehips and bioflavonoids.

KEY TO SUPPLEMENTS: COVER ALL BASES

In your daily food supplement, you are buttressing any deficiencies which may be in your diet. It is preposterous to suppose that every bite of food should be chemically analyzed for contents.

Again, who cares where and how deficiency may exist?

Sometimes you can't eat right. You will be in a hurry and have to stop off somewhere for lunch. You can't make a research-project out of which restaurant, or just where you're least likely to pick up salmonella. You have to grab a bite and run.

Or you may do it by choice. It's fun to have a quick lunch with friends or, as a loner, try a new diner.

But you can't expect to meet all your food requirements while eating on the run.

So here's how you cover yourself:

2 BASIC RULES OF FOOD SUPPLEMENTS

There are two basic rules which cover everything:

1. Buy the best, top-quality, complex vitamin-mineral supplement, containing as many different food factors as possible. Read labels. Taking charge of

your own case is your "yellow brick road" to better health than you have ever known--and, with that, a stronger, happier, healthier heart.

There are many different kinds of food supplements. We strongly advise you to go to a health-food store, not just a drugstore, and read labels and make comparisons right there in the store. Ask questions.

Some supplements are made with a real-foods basis. Some contain food andherb concentrates, which not only nourish you, but help to cleanse the liver, thus helping to reestablish your native ability to make your own lecithin and protect your heart.

You will find heart formulae which also contain herbs, minerals. Some formulations wisely and conveniently provide a.m. supplements and p.m. supplements. Why wisely? Because your body uses certain kinds of nutrition for waking hours, and sleep utilizes and requires different kinds.

Many people buy separate vitamins, minerals, herbs, enzymes, and co-enzymes, and make up their own day and night packets.

To search out the full blessings of these wonderful alternatives, enjoy full complexity by changing around until you hit on the combination that suits you best. And you'll know, too. We tend to forget that, after all, the heart is right here--in me, in you. You know your heart pretty well. You know your body better than anybody alive.

Often better than the most sophisticated medical diagnostic tests. Why do we say this? Because expensive, intrusive and often painful tests can produce errors that can be disastrous. Even the august Journal of the American Medical Association has published the disturbing fact that 27% of clinical tests are in error because of faulty instruments--that's a nation-wide average.

When you wake up in the morning, your good guess is probably better than that!

We're not suggesting that you not consult a physician if in serious difficulties, physically, and avail yourself of modern diagnostic medicine (as we said in Chapter Three). But do remember than when you turn your health over to somebody else, he or she is one step removed from your own body. You are closer than that person is. Repeatedly, week after week, we work with people who have been badly diagnosed and destructively prescribed.

The solution? As said above, the first rule is to cover all basis.

The second rule is this:

2. Feed like to like, food and supplement.

This produces amazing results. If you are fighting infection and choose to emphasize vitamin C, also increase those foods containing C naturally. If you need extra protein, don't settle for protein supplements only, increase natural protein--something that has lived, like beef or soy beans.

Certainly, many supplements are manufactured from live food sources. But to these concentrated forms, add the untampered, unconcentrated, undamaged form, because it will bring into your body the complex, surrounding food factors which make the supplement work better.

In the feeding of any gland or organ, try to find the tissue of that gland or organ in a reliable health food store. For the heart, eat dehydrated heart tissue, and also eat real beef heart in small amounts (if pos-

sible, swallow 1/4 cup of this, raw, with a small toma-
to-juice chaser).

The primary food for the thyroid gland is--how
simple can it be?--thyroid tissue. You don't need a prescription, you need a health food store and a little
ready cash.

THE THYROID, VITAMIN A AND
BETA-CAROTEN

This prescription applies to all vitamins. For
instance, for vitamin A, you should seek out this vitamin in its non-isolated form, as a portion of sauteed
liver and/or dark green leaves of any kind. If your thyroid gland is the least faulty, you may not be able to
convert beta-carotene into A efficiently, so do not
assume that ample beta-carotene is providing you
with sufficient A.

Often we encounter people who are taking beta-
carotene, and upon investigation, find that they are
not utilizing it. They remain seriously low in A and are
extremely puzzled by this. A failure such as this
endangers the heart for so many reasons, both direct
and indirect.

Only when the thyroid gland is working perfectly,
is it useful and non-dangerous to eat isolated beta-
carotene. This is something to find out about yourself,
for a fact. No "opinions" allowable here. If your thyroid
is malfunctioning, or your basal-metabolism is down
even one degree, you will have better luck to provide
your beta-carotene, precursor of A, from whole foods.
Then, when your thyroid is perfectly normalized, the
supplement will work for you.

These are reasons, as you can plainly see, why you should read about these matters for yourself. They are all easy to understand once you have brushed over them a few times, and you can trust your own judgment increasingly as you take intelligent steps toward health on your own.

RECAPPING THE BASICS OF FOOD SUPPLEMENTS

In brief, the two basic steps to assure yourself of sound nutrition and to make food-supplements work best for your heart, are:

1. Use the most complete, complex food supplement of the highest quality you can afford. Rely on it and enjoy it. Also, consider a thorough a.m.-p.m. formula to make waking up and going to sleep an enhanced pleasure and health gain.

You may have health reasons (discussed separately in several places) for increasing, say, vitamin B-3--niacin. Or you wish to increase stamina and well-being, and opt for B-1 and B-5. These, you can add above and beyond your daily multiple dosage, in which case, you should--

2. Emphasize whole foods which contain the same vitamins and/or minerals you have chosen to increase.

You will have health reasons of your own. When you increase individual nutrients to meet your special needs, it's best to buttress these additions with the complex, surrounding food factors and enzymes which no food supplement can completely contain. We mean plain food here. Use your daily meals to reinforce your own particular vitamin-mineral intake. In the battle for greatest ease, satisfaction, practical results and supreme complexity of the wonderful micro-nutrients, this is your best bet.

CHEAPEST HEART MEDICINE

For years doctors have pooh-poohed the beneficial effects of vitamin E (see item below), but, thankfully, their numbers are getting fewer every year. In fact, the doubters and scoffers are definitely in the scientific rear-guard.

Studies continue to show that long-term use of vitamin E lowers the incidence of heart disease. It accomplishes this "miracle" by reducing platelet adhesion--and fibrous plaque on arterial walls--thus returning abnormal platelets to normality. This keeps the blood free-flowing, so coronaries are reduced.

One long-term study, published in the American Journal of Clinical Pathology, concluded that vitamin E helps anti-clotting, improves oxygen utilization, and even controls the patch-scar that replaces damaged heart tissue, while improving capillary permeability.

How much E is enough? A reasonable daily dose for those seeking coronary disease protection is 400 IU (International Units)--up to 800 IU daily.

Of course, some old-line medical sources continue to claim that dietary sources of E (and other vitamins) are amply sufficient. But facts don't support that. In a definitive Harvard School of Public Health study of coronary heart disease, those with E solely from food did not experience the protective effect as those who took vitamin E supplements.

Those who took the highest amount of E experienced a statistically significant 32% to 34% reduction in coronary disease risk.

Note: For maximum effect, the antioxidant mineral selenium should be taken in conjunction with E. (See "Update on Antioxidants" below.) Reasonable daily amounts of selenium are 50 micrograms for protection and 100 mcg. daily for control.

For further corroboration: In April, 1996, British researchers reported that daily vitamin E pills seem to reduce heart attacks 75% when taken by people with bad hearts.

FEEDING FRENZY ON VITAMIN E

With all this increasing clinical evidence on the health value of Vitamin E (and other antioxidants), many health-food stores have even experienced shortages in the product, or at least had trouble keeping E stocked on their shelves.

And not just independent stores have been vitamin-E-deficient. General Nutrition, the nation's largest vitamin and health-food chain, actually had some of earnings reports fall below analysts' expectations because of worldwide shortages of E. (Synthetic vitamin E, made from chemicals, has not been in short supply, since it's less in demand.)

In addition to demand, some of the periodic shortages can be traced to poor soybean crops and problems at Archer-Daniels-Midland Co. This giant agribusiness is one of the largest suppliers of raw vitamin E, which is extracted from the distillate left over from the manufacture of soy and other vegetable oils. The raw liquid vitamin E is then shipped to vitamin makers, who put it into capsule form.

Helping the makers of vitamin E supplements is an absence of side effects and the fact that recent studies say a daily vitamin-E dosage of 100 to 400 IUs is needed to reap its benefits--far more than can be consumed in a normal diet.

Vitamin E's move into the consumer mainstream would have stunned early researchers, who fought many naysayers. Among these pioneers were two Canadian doctors, Evan Shute and his brother Wilfrid, who treated heart patients with vitamin E in the late 1940s at their clinic in London, Ontario. Both were denounced throughout the medical profession.

Denham Harman, a University of Nebraska medical professor, provided the theoretical framework that explained why Vitamin E worked against free radicals in the 1950s. "People paid no attention," the doctor recalled. "This went up into the '60s and '70s. It was extremely difficult to get any money to do the work. All of a sudden things were different."

UPDATE ON ANTIOXIDANTS

Antioxidants vitamins have a number of beneficial effects in the fight against heart disease. As mentioned above, vitamin E is known to make platelets less sticky, thus protecting against the formation of harmful clots. It also increases HDL levels and protects the other antioxidants. And vitamin E has been used successfully to treat claudication, a problem of atherosclerotic plaque blocking the arteries to the legs.

Vitamin C also helps decrease platelet stickiness, while strengthening the arterial walls against damage, increasing HDL levels and lowering the mortality from heart attacks.

The mineral selenium is considered an antioxidant, because it's necessary for the proper function of the important antioxidant enzyme glutathione peroxidase (which renders harmless the oxidized lipids called lipid peroxides). Low selenium levels are associated with high rates of atherosclerotic heart disease. Selenium also makes the platelets less sticky.

Zinc is also needed for antioxidant enzymes to function, and also makes platelets less sticky. However, in moderate-to-high doses (above 50 milligrams a day), it will lower HDLs (the good cholesterol). This is probably due to the fact that zinc competes with copper, which seems to aid in lowering cholesterol and strengthening the connective tissue in the artery wall. Thus, people taking zinc supplementation for various reasons (prostate, skin, and immune function, for example) should always take copper as well.

ENERGY COCKTAIL--REBUILD YOUR ADRENALS

If you're low on energy, you may learn that your adrenal glands are as tired as you are. Unfortunately, this is often the case.

One frequent reason is the avoidance of eggs, which has become almost axiomatic as "progressive" the last twenty-five years.

Yet egg lecithin (if the eggs are cooked easy, not hard) is a prime food for nourishing and restoring those exhausted adrenal glands. The small amount of salt you may wish for your eggs is also an adrenal food.

But so are vitamins B-5 (pantothenic acid) and C.

So, above your daily supplements, you may wish to emphasize the nutrients just mentioned. Doing so will help to rebuild your adrenal glands, ease stress on your heart (B-5 is a main anti-stress food) and provide surprising, new energy.

Now here is where our example pays off:

To support B-5, add its main source food, royal jelly, to your diet. This is a splendid secret. The small female bee larva begins with a brief destiny of five weeks. That's her expected lifespan. By five or six weeks she will literally fly her wings off.

But then, if she is chosen to be their queen, the bees will feed her royal jelly. She will ingest rich sources of vitamin B-5. Her lifespan will increase from those brief five or six weeks to well over five years, even up to nine years.

When you increase B-5, increase some meal-time source food. This will add the unknowns, all kinds of precious micro-nutrients, and the surrounding food factors.

VITAMINS AND SOURCE FOODS

It's simple but critical enough to bear another repetition: Just consider which nutrient (if any) you wish to increase for your own, particular reasons. To make these added vitamins or minerals or co-factors serve you especially well, and to prolong their effects, increase the source foods of those same nutrients.

Examples:

Co-enzyme Q-10 is found in beef heart (raw) and golden corn (raw).

Vitamin C is found in citrus fruit of all kinds, in red peppers, including the very hot pepper, cayenne.

When you increase iron, eat a few raisins along with it, to supply unknowns and complexity.

When you use additional A, increase your fish consumption, beef liver and/or dark green vegetables. This will not cause you to get too much of the particular nutrient.

Indeed, the complex sources, providing nature's choice of surrounding food factors, tend to protect you from excess.

Once you have tried these ideas a few times, you will wonder how you ever got along without them. And of course, your health--and particularly heart health--will rise. You may even find yourself singing.

Notes

_____

_____

_____

_____

_____

_____

_____

XI. B VITAMINS TO THE RESCUE

ALWAYS ENRICH B VITAMINS WITH B-SOURCE FOODS

When you increase any separate B vitamin, always increase your B-vitamin source foods. It is not necessary to eat every one of these at every meal. But supply your kitchen with them and use them as staples for heart health and long life:

Nine sources of main "B-foods":

1. Brewer's yeast--look for the kind with enzymes included, and try several for taste. (This yeast is not the kind used in baking bread.)

2. Yogurt--use the plain kind, without commercially added fruit. This will also provide friendly bacteria by the billion, which you need in your intestinal tract. Fresh yogurt will help to implant these bacteria in small and large intestines and offset the toxins which we have discussed as leading to liver-poisoning and the loss of its lecithin production. Yes, this B-source food can also be considered, indirectly, as a heart food.

3. Raw wheat germ--nearly 80 percent of the fat in

wheat germ-the sprouting part of the wheat kernel--is unsaturated, the kind proven to help reduce "bad" LDL cholesterol. Further, wheat germ is brimming with vitamin E.

Wheat germ is also rich in folate, a B vitamin vital to the production of new blood cells, and magnesium, which may help protect your heart, arteries and blood pressure.

But--wouldn't you know?--the very life-giving germ of the wheat is exactly what millers remove to make a "simplified" starch for baking devitalized breads. Does this sound familiar? It should. The simplified bread is a kind of robbery, and, of course, we are back to our perennial theme of complexity. The wheat germ is the complex part of the grain. Naturally, it's the best part.

This raw food requires refrigeration and should be kept as much from air as possible until used up.

You can use wheat germ to add flavor-and crunch-to virtually any dish, from cereal to meat loaf. Wheat germ has an appealing nutty taste, and is so versatile that you can use it in almost anything. Here are some ways to add it to your diet:

* In making muffins, substitute 1/2 cup of wheat germ for 1/2 cup of flour. Note: Wheat germ tends to absorb moisture in baked goods, so add one to two table-spoons of water per 1/2 cup of wheat germ.

* Use wheat germ in cake and bread mixes. Replace no more than a third of the flour with wheat germ, however. It doesn't contain much gluten, the stuff that helps bread rise.

* Sprinkle wheat germ on cold or hot cereal. You can add the wheat germ while hot cereal is cooking or just before eating. Or mix wheat germ into low-fat or nonfat yogurt or low-fat or nonfat vanilla, rice or tapioca pudding.

* Sprinkle wheat germ on tossed salads. Or try topping cooked vegetables with a blend of wheat germ and a drop of olive oil.

* Mix a small amount of wheat germ into meatloaf.

4. Raw nuts, especially almonds. The thin, tan-colored skin on the almond is a rare source of B-17, a vitamin which you will not find in any B-complex supplement. The reason: B-17 is a form of cyanide!

Take your daily cyanide only in natural form, please. There's no danger. Just don't eat an entire cupful of apple seeds; this is an example of a raw food which can be, in ridiculously huge amounts, dangerous, even fatal.

Almonds are also loaded with calcium, vitamin E and magnesium, which helps regulate blood pressure. Almonds, and nuts in general, are also high in monounsaturated fat, which has been shown to lower total and LDL cholesterol without detrimentally affecting HDL cholesterol. Nearly two-thirds (65 percent) of the total fat of almonds is monounsaturated.

Researchers at Loma Linda University in Loma Linda, California, examined the link between eating nuts--including almonds, walnuts and peanuts--and a reduced risk of heart disease in more than 31,000 Seventh-Day Adventists. The researchers found that those who ate nuts more than four times a week had about half the risk of suffering a heart attack (fatal or nonfatal) of those who ate nuts less than once a week.

An ounce of almonds (20 to 25 nuts) contains about 170 calories--not exactly a low-calorie snack. But folks who add almonds to their diets often find that their weight stays the same, probably because as they eat more almonds, they tend to cut down on other foods and replace animal protein with plant protein.

Raw cashews are also one of our rare food-sources of vitamin D. Sunflower seeds and pumpkin seeds offer the advantage of being perfect foods. There are oils in these nuts, and oils can become rancid. Therefore, in all raw grains, seeds and nuts, purchase only the fresh, and keep them cold until eaten.

While most people enjoy roasted cashews, more oil will have been added in the roasting and, when baked--there you are, stuck with more heat-damaged oil. So learn to enjoy the flavor and perfection of the raw. Also, many people find that cashews, the roasted kind, give them flatulence. These folks often absorb the raw cashews will less difficulty.

If chewing is difficult, toss 1/4 cup of any combination of these nuts into your blender and add to soups (don't actually cook them with the soup, add when served), drinks, warm raw milk at bedtime or as topping for fresh salads.

Again, don't worry about the oil. It is not much, and when the nuts and seeds are not old (rancid), the oils are excellent for digestion, for your gallbladder and for your body cells. (When oils are severely limited in the diet, the gallbladder cannot form gall to digest oils. Result: Improperly digested oils can't enter cells, and nourishment is harmed.) Walnuts: Just as with almonds, an ounce of walnuts contains about 180 calories and 17 grams of fat. But eaten in moderation, walnuts may actually help lower your blood cholesterol without ballooning your waistline.

How? The answer lies in the type of fat this nut contains. Seventy percent of the fat in walnuts is polyunsaturated. In fact, one study found the ratio of polyunsaturated to saturated fat is 7 to 1--one of the highest amongnaturally occurring foods.

Walnuts are also rich in linolenic acid, an omega-3 fatty acid, also found in canola oil. In fact, this is similar to the cholesterol-lowering omega-3's found in fatty fish.

Recommendation: Eat walnuts in place of, not in addition to, other fats--especially saturated fats. Try these nutty serving suggestions.

* Sprinkle chopped shelled walnuts over steamed brussels sprouts or baked sweet potatoes.

* Toss a small amount of chopped walnuts into a salad. The nuts will add flavor, texture and vitamin E.

* Add chopped walnuts to pancake batter.

* If you have a food processor, make walnut sprinkles. Mix 1 cup of ground shelled walnuts with 1/2 cup of bread crumbs, then bake at 325 degrees for about 15 minutes, or until the sprinkles are crisp and golden brown. Stir in 1/2 teaspoon of cayenne pepper and one tablespoon of paprika, then cool. Use the sprinkles on salads, soups or pasta, in place of Parmesan cheese.

5. Raw root vegetables provide B vitamins otherwise missing in your diet and are major B-source foods.

Root vegetables include garlic, onion, potato, radish, turnip, carrot--anything that grows underground.

Note: the important vitamin B-12 grows primarily in soil that has not been treated with weed killer, crop dusting or commercial fertilizers. This B-12, growing well and spontaneously in organic soil, will, along the food chain, appear in crops which send their roots into it, and thence into cattle, and next in the diet of humans which eat those crops and/or beef.

Root vegetables grown in such fine soil actually absorb nutrients of high quality into their skins, and thus, larger carrots, pound for pound, contain more nutrition than tender young carrots which have not been in the ground long.

These foods, far from being poisoned by the earth in which they've grown, have become important food sources for health-minded people. If such root vegetables have grown in pesticide- and weed-killer-free soil, wash them as little as possible. Indeed, it is even wholesome not to wash them at all, wiping away any grit or brushing them with a damp towel--and then eating them, directly.

It would seem superfluous to say that to peel such foods is just one more simplification of the complex and wonderful. (Note: Jicama may require partial skinning, and garlic must be virtually shelled.)

Grating raw potato onto salads, or adding thin-sliced raw radish, turnip and parsnip on the plate makes a nice garnish, tasty and wholesome. Small cubes of raw jicama and potato may be tossed into green salads, and even into potato salad with the cooked portion of the potato.

Caution: Raw beets, when eaten in quantity, can make the throat feel "coughy." Straight beet juice will certainly do this, so grate only small amounts of this rich food into salad or other dishes.

Even so, do not peel before cooking. Include several inches of beet tops, cover with good water and simmer slowly. During the last half-hour of cooking, you may wish to add onion and cabbage for a richer final borscht. Slip peel the beets and reserve the deep red "meat" for many uses in salads, eaten alone with a dressing or served hot with a touch of butter and white pepper. Immediately blend the dross, cabbage, onion, beet skin, tops and all, with the cooking water, and strain, as your base for homemade beet borscht. You will find grit in this, so remove it carefully.

6. Liver--any kind (except polar bear!), cooked, though fresh beef liver can be diced and swallowed raw, without chewing. (We're not the first to recommend this, and, no, it's not a fraternity hazing!) In any case, this is a prime source of B vitamins, helping to support the individual B vitamins you may wish to take. Never overcook this delicate food.

(White onions and green bell pepper, sauteed before putting fillets in pan, provide a flavor that mitigates the taste of liver, which some people do not enjoy. In fact, most organ meats are made more pleasing by some taste-factor in the cooked, green pepper.)

7. Whole grains of all kinds--for the same reasons that wheat germ is good: the unmilled grains are complex, having everything the way nature designed them. While these require cooking or soaking, they can be sprouted, too. They also are available ground into fine flours for baking, adding to soups and many dishes. In all cases, avoid overcooking these perfect foods.

Whole-grain flours can be slightly toasted and added to beverages and soups.

8. Whey, a by-product of butter- and cheese-making. This is an amazing food, contains original B vitamins, a few not found in most other foods; and the protein is one of the best you will find. If milk sugar (lactose) is not a problem for you, you will find many uses for this superior food.

There is a story about an old English gentleman many years ago who lived in a cottage by himself, maintaining his cow and a small vegetable garden. He milked his cow, making butter and cheese, which he sold to neighbors as his livelihood.

Being poor, he drank the by-products of his trade, the whey. It was left over, and nobody wanted it. He couldn't pour it out, so he drank it. It was perhaps the staple of his simple diet, including also his organic vegetables, which he fertilized well.

He lived to be above 120 years (or so the story goes). He was such an amazing fellow, he was invited into London to visit the queen. There, on rich court foods, the fellow's health failed, and, in a few weeks, he died.

Such instances are, of course, anecdotal, and scientists discard real-life instances with a frightening haste and thoroughness. Yet those interested in health may find the little story of merit. Whey, I think, and a little garden of organic vegetables, may be what the tale is about. In that sense it is a true story, and is not the only account of long life amid simple living.

From our point of view, his diet was quite the opposite of "simple." The rich foods in the London court were simple. They had been baked, boiled, fried, sauced, ground, rebaked and richly seasoned, to say nothing of wined and brandied. These exotic and sophisticated processes were not making their complex dishes complex foods, but, by methodical degrees, killing off everything, making the complex into the simple and turning good food into useless, spicy carbon.

Meanwhile, all those years, the elderly gentleman had been enjoying complex combinations of enzymes, co enzymes, vitamins, minerals and all the unknown food factors of which nature was capable. For this gent, his journey to London was, we regret to say, a step down.

Try to find your whey packaged so as to exclude light of any kind. Light destroys some B vitamins. This food also, when the package is opened, should be resealed and kept cold until used.

9. Small amounts of blackstrap molasses. This interesting food is, once again, the "dross" removed to make simple table sugar, a thoroughly devitalized food.

And where has the vitality of the original sugar-beets gone? Into that dark, pungent syrup, the very essence of the source food from which the sugar has been made.

Blackstrap molasses has been, over the years, such a drug on the market that tons of it are sold cheaply to cattlemen, who pour this by-product of the sugar industry onto dry fodder to replace the damage of crop-dusting, commercial fertilizers, the lack of green fodder and even, perhaps, the lack of exercise. Cattle, au naturale, do move around. They do seem to like to walk, though ranchers don't like their steers to walk much, as it loses pounds of salable weight, requires more watering and may make the cuts of beef tough, because of the additional musculature.

Tsk, tsk--devitalized cows? Who need more exercise than they're getting? And require food supplements, just like you and me? Yes! For the ranchers must boost their cows' vitamins, you see, to make cows they can sell.

Further, the animal metabolism absolutely does require all the nutrients for supporting life. Deprived of necessary nutrition, even cows get heart attacks! When ranchers cut back too far on good food, the cows literally drop dead in the field.

Well, so do people, don't they? And for the exact

same reasons, every step of the way.

The blackstrap molasses, however, still contains rich sugars, and so this food should be used only in small amounts. It supplies one more very useful source for the full group of B's.

Small amounts can be put into children's drinks when they don't, won't or can't take usual supplements, and it can be used moderately in cooking. It's not bad at all in a cup of warm milk at bedtime.

This again is a food which you might have in your kitchen, and never have considered as a B-vitamin source food.

Note: Sorghum isn't the same as blackstrap.

SEARCH OUT MORE SOURCES OF B VITAMINS YOURSELF

The nine foods listed above should suggest larger categories, comprising dozens of foods, many kinds of raw nuts, all sorts of grains and root vegetables. But look elsewhere, too, as there are many other sources.

WARD OFF HEART DISEASE (AND VAMPIRES)

Garlic is not a vice, no matter how pungent and sinful it may seem. Numerous studies indicate that garlic may help overpower high cholesterol levels (as well as warding off vampires, according to Transylvanian legend).

Garlic contains allicin, a compound activated when the bulb is cut, crushed or cooked. When allicin, which contains sulfur, reacts with oxygen, it breaks down into other compounds that give garlic its distinctive odor and provide its apparent cholesterol-busting abilities.

Garlic also seems to keep blood platelets from clumping, preventing clots that could trigger heart attack or stroke. Garlic may also stimulate the blood's natural clot-dissolving processes, which helps get rid of clots that do form.

Researchers at Tulane University School of Medicine in New Orleans gave 42 men and women with elevated cholesterol either 900 milligrams of garlic extract (divided among three capsules) or a placebo every day, After 12 weeks, the total cholesterol of those taking the garlic extract fell 6 percent, and their LDL cholesterol plunged 11 percent. By contrast, the total and LDL cholesterol of those consuming the placebo fell only 1 and 3 percent, respectively.

In one European study, 40 patients with high cholesterol consumed either 900 milligrams of garlic powder or a placebo every day for 16 weeks. The total cholesterol of the garlic powder group fell an average of 21 percent, while their triglycerides--another blood fat implicated in heart disease--fell 24 percent. The total cholesterol of those taking the placebo declined only 3 percent, while their triglycerides fell 5 percent.

Of course, this aromatic herb is popular for other than health reasons.

Americans consume about 250 million pounds of it annually. But 0 people took a placebo. Not only did the garlic-eaters' cholesterol levels fall an average of 9 percent, their risk of dying or of having a second heart attack declined as %,ell. The cholesterol of the individuals taking the placebo didn't change.

New And Natural Ways To Your Lower Blood Pressure, Cholesterol And Stress

Medical researchers aren't sure how much garlic is needed to reduce cholesterol levels. One Dutch study concluded that it would take 7 to 28 cloves of garlic a day to help curb cholesterol. But a more recent U.S. study indicates significantly smaller doses of garlic may do some good.

And you don't need to consume pounds of pungent cloves. You can try garlic supplements--odorless pills and powders created to offer the health benefits of garlic without offending those around you.

If you do like to use garlic in cooking, however, one of the easiest ways is to chop it, crush it and saute it in a little olive or canola oil. Then you can add it to soups, stews and many other dishes. Or add ground fresh garlic to salad dressings and marinades.

But if you'd prefer not to handle fresh garlic, use commercially prepared garlic paste or minced garlic in oil. Or try garlic powder (made from dehydrated and pulverized cloves), garlic oil (distilled from cloves) or aged garlic extract (a water-based garlic product). One large garlic clove is equal to 1/2 teaspoon of garlic powder and 1 teaspoon of minced garlic.

Garlic supplements are available in health food stores and most drugstores. One popular formulation, Kwai powder tablets, contains the equivalent of 2.7 grams of fresh garlic in each 900-milligram dose. One clove of garlic equals about 3 grams of fresh garlic.

Warnings: Avoid garlic salt, which can be loaded with sodium and have the health benefits of fresh garlic. You should also know that, consumed in large amounts, garlic can cause a variety of side effects, including heartburn, gas, skin irritation and allergic reactions. Cooking garlic tends to weaken such irritating properties.

And if you're taking blood-thinning drugs, you should

consult your physician before consuming garlic or garlic supplements. Reason: garlic has been shown to delay blood-clotting time.

HOW ENZYMES AND HORMONES WORK TOGETHER

We could call this "The Fine Art of Eating." Much of what could be said under this heading you already know, and so we shall not linger too long. Of course, you were told as a child to chew your food well. "Don't bolt your food!" some parent probably said periodically, especially just before playtime.

But the meal actually begins with anticipation. You know (even if you haven't heard of Pavlov) that enzymes begin to develop and stir at the mere smell of good food cooking. Even foods not so beneficial--coffee brewing, bacon frying--can stir the sense of hunger and desire.

But as to your heart, this "fine art of eating" is truly essential, as you'll see.

Whole books have been written on this topic, books on food combining, adjusting your acid/alkaline balance with foods, foods for cleansing the system, foods for wholesome dieting and fasting--endless books telling you what and how to eat!

We shall duplicate as little of these fine volumes as possible (though we recommend you read them when you can). But we cannot pass by without sharing with you an important point about, say, your steak dinner. It has a direct bearing on two wonderful things:

1. food enjoyment, and

2. your heart.

Yes, they do go together.

But first we must touch very briefly on the basics of chewing--as if you haven't been told a hundred times how to do it. But perhaps you will find something new here:

WHICH FOODS REQUIRE MORE CHEWING, WHICH LESS?

You've probably heard the old saw: "Drink your solids, chew your liquids." Quaint. Even helpful. But not exact.

Raw foods and starches require maximum work in the mouth. Raw foods--fruits and vegetables--contain a great deal of fiber, which must be crushed if your system is to get the benefit. Moreover, these plus the starchy foods, breads and grains, from dinner rolls to corn chips, must become thoroughly alkaline in your mouth, before swallowing.

Your saliva must prepare fruit, raw vegetables and starches for the stomach. Otherwise, the stomach, confronted with improperly delivered food, will commence to find ways to hurry them along, force them from the stomach insufficiently digested. It's not uncommon for these good foods to cause stomachache and, of course, inevitably, loss of food value.

Yet always remember: you don't get away with it free. You pay for every bite. You spend your internal resources: enzymes, hormones and finally friendly bacteria, plus precious fluids of all kinds, to process food whether or not it really feeds you. Every time such foods get wasted, you still pay.

But then, meats, eggs, cheese, milk, and even legumes: beans, peas, garbanzos (chick peas), black-eyed peas; and nuts of all kinds do not require such patient grinding away with the molars. These are high protein foods, and your hydrochloric acid will digest them far more efficiently than your attempts to turn them into bolus in the mouth and chyle further down.

Beans and cheese, eggs--these protein foods can be chewed until essentially smooth, if lumpy, and swallowed.

HOW TO DIGEST A STEAK

Meat, however, requires very strong hydrochloric acid--a powerful digestant--and this brings us to your own digestive system, and what happens with your steak. You recall our discussion of the danger of red meats decaying in the lower intestines?

Well, here is one more method to cope with that problem.

There are three foods which set the stage for a nice, broiled steak--the steak is not one of them. These foods, or any one of them, is what you should eat or sip slowly before the main course:

1. Fresh fruit;

2. Vegetable soup;

3. A meat bouillon or broth.

Fresh fruit cup as an appetizer. This isn't a side dish to the steak. It is a course to be served and enjoyed before the main course.

Since citrus fruits turn to an alkaline ash in the stomach, these might be replaced to greater advantage with other ripe fruits--pineapple, mango, papaya, grapes, peaches, pears and so on.

As just mentioned, because these fruits contain high fiber, they should be chewed slowly and enjoyed.

Or your first course can be soup.

On a cold day you might prefer a hot soup composed of several kinds of slowly simmered (not heavily boiled) vegetables. The broth should not be opaque with cheese, thickened with starch or tangy with spice, but tasty. Use the milder Italian spices which compliment vegetable flavors.

Even better: add a soupbone to the broth, or diced chicken breast.

But possibly the best pre-beef course is, surprisingly, meat broth. This can be a prepared bouillon, or an almost clear chicken broth, or very slowly simmered shank. But, in all cases, remove the cooked fat, leaving the straight extraction from the meat.

This is the beginning of a very surprising process. For all three--the well-chewed fresh fruit, the vegetable soup and the meat broth--belong to a special category of food called extractive substances.

HOW EXTRACTIVES HELP DIGESTION

Fruit, soup or bouillon are not marinades to be poured over your steak. Nor are they a solution in which your eaten steak is set afloat, while your stomach tries to decide what to do about it.

No, these foods serve a different, more intriguing, even mysterious purpose. As extractives they trigger a hormone in the lower portion of your stomach.

Now remember, hormones are primarily messengers. And this hormone, secretin, leaves immediately to inform the bloodstream. Secretin enters the bloodstream, circulates to all bodily organs, perhaps to spread the good news that help is coming.

This hormone then re-enters the stomach, but now at the upper end. At this point enzymes having directly to do with the foods eaten begin to flow.

But most important of all, because of this hormone, great quantities of hydrochloric acid begin to flow in readiness for real meat, complete proteins--this is a meal that will digest very well indeed.

Yet, people often believe that a great green salad, which is chomped a little, but not carefully chewed, will do the same thing. It doesn't. Neither do vast quantities of drink--whiskey, wine, beer. And why? Because none of these are extractive substances, literally, the extracted juices of fruit, vegetable or meat.

Note: these three special foods are not grains, nuts, dairy or oils. As special substances, they truly serve a unique function.

It is wonderful, we think, that the body really does know what to do with food, and eagerly will do everything possible for you, if but given the chance.

The Chinese have known all about this trick for helping the body to digest meats for centuries. It will work for you, too, and for anyone who views the fine art of eating not as a pigpen affair, but as one of life's splendid ceremonies, the purely beneficent banquet.

XII: THE BEST HEART MEDICINE?

NIACIN MAY BE THE BEST PREVENTATIVE

Niacin (nicotinic acid) is vitamin B-3, and is the antidote to the disease pellagra. While pellagra is endemic to parts of the world--like Asia and the southeastern United States--niacin today is used mainly for general nutritional purposes, somewhat for athletic purposes, even as a sexual stimulant; for treating schizophrenia and MÇniäre's syndrome (affecting the inner ear and sense of balance).

Its widest present use, however, is in lowering blood pressure in heart patients and, to an equal degree, in lowering cholesterol; though the effect of this unusual vitamin in lowering blood pressure does not seem to be caused entirely by its cholesterol-lowering properties.

Extremely high blood pressures have successfully, safely, and even quickly been lowered by the use of vitamin B-3 when cholesterol was apparently not the problem, and indeed, pressure is often lowered before cholesterol, or plaque deposits in arteries, is significantly reduced. In fact, when given in sufficient doses, niacin can reduce total cholesterol, elevate HDL cholesterol and significantly reduce triglyceride levels. (See niacin-cholesterol test below.)

Thus, the vitamin appears to have two distinct capacities, though both afflictions treated seem usually to coincide in the same person.

THE AMA GETS ON THE NIACIN BANDWAGON

The mainstream medical establishment is finally getting around to admitting the advantages of prescribing niacin for heart patients. As the Harvard Heart Letter pointed out, this B vitamin is natural, proven effective and inexpensive--three important criteria that few medications can meet.

The Harvard Heart Letter comes right out with the truth: that niacin can reduce the risk of coronary artery disease when taken in much larger doses than the recommended daily allowance of 15-20 mg. In fact, they conclude that niacin is probably the most effective available drug for raising HDL cholesterol levels. Here is a "drug," as they perversely call it, which costs less than one-tenth the price of "alternative medications" that reduce blood-cholesterol levels. Moreover, many expert medical panels and managed-care organizations are now encouraging physicians and their patients with high cholesterol to try niacin first if dietary and lifestyle modifications are not successful. Here's one reason for the medical establishment's belated endorsement of this miracle vitamin.

BREAKTHROUGH NIACIN-CHOLESTEROL STUDY

In one study of middle-aged men with low HDL-cholesterol levels, volunteers were assigned to take regular niacin for 12 weeks and no treatment for another 12 weeks. The niacin dosage began at 125 mg three times a day and doubled each week for the next two weeks. The dose was progressively increased to a maximum of 3,000 mg per day. To stay in the study, patients had to be able to tolerate at least 1,500 mg per day.

Among the patients in the study who were able to use the high-dose niacin, HDL (the good) cholesterol rose by 31% from an average of 32 mg/dl.

LDL cholesterol fell from 123 mg/dl to 101 mg/dl (an 18% decrease). The ratio of total to HDL cholesterol declined from 6 (with a total cholesterol of 192 and an HDL of 31.7) to 4 (total cholesterol of 165 and an HDL of 42). Niacin also decreased average triglyceride levels from 197 mg/dl to 119 mg/dl.

These improvements in lipid profile distinctly lower the risk for coronary artery disease. And the clinical researchers stressed that no other class of cholesterol-reducing drug has this full range of beneficial effects.

The medical establishment--not wanting to go over- board in their enthusiasm, mind you--concludes that niacin is mainly advisable for people with a low HDL-cholesterol level and elevated LDL-cholesterol and triglyceride levels. Niacin, they say, is also "worth considering" for people with a normal total-cholesterol level but a low HDL-cholesterol level.

Why isn't it worth considering for everybody?

HOW NIACIN WORKS ITS MIRACLES

Niacin has the unique ability to dilate capillaries, physically restoring vast amounts of the lost bloodstream which so frequently accompany a rise in pressure.

As capillaries re-open, admitting blood into blood-starved tissues, nothing less than miles of "watercourse" are regained for the bed of arterialblood.

Certainly, in most patients, elevated pressure can be accounted for by constrictions, which are even apparent to the eye, as well as under the microscope. In turn, the opening of capillary passages is visible also by the characteristic flushing of the skin, turning pallid complexions pink, not unlike a sunburn; and the sensation of the flushing is almost precisely that of sunburn, as well.

With the flow of fresh blood into narrowed passages, a tingling is usually felt, reaching in some cases a fever pitch, a burning sensation. In rarer cases, the person experiences a rash, which is not exactly the same as benign flushing and which sometimes remains after the "niacin effect" has subsided. In such case, caution should be used not to aggravate a complicating condition.

Peculiarly, the flushing or sunburn sensation is as frequently disliked by women as it is enjoyed by men, who often like the heat, a stimulation to the musculature. This has led to niacin's use in gymnasiums by bodybuilders who want to retain a warm "pump" or engorgement of blood through maximum contractions of their muscles.

Muscle strength reaches its peak at maximum saturation of blood within the tissues, and inasmuch as niacin dilates capillaries, it assists in maintaining this peak.

Since weight training is usually done in "reps" and "sets," there are delays in continuing even a rapid workout. Yet in a busy gym, bodybuilders sometimes have to wait to use popular equipment. This delay, not always brief, can work against peak performance, by constituting a cooling down of the muscles. Thus niacin helps to bridge necessary rest periods and unplanned delays.

THE TRUTH ABOUT NIACIN AND THE LIVER

By 1985, the popularity of this vitamin for gymnasium use had reached a peak--just as the suspicion that high niacin intake damaged the liver began to quell the enthusiasm of athletes.

Then, Dr. Abram Hoffer, who had used nicotinic acid (niacin) in psychiatric work and research as early as 1955, disclosed in 1990 that the alterations in the liver were wrongly identified changes in enzymes, not damage. The furor had been for nothing.

To date, Hoffer's niacin update has not been refuted, and yet you will hear the same "flaw" repeated with the same peculiar persistency which has haunted vitamin C and other profoundly useful nutrients. You will read, for instance, that niacin causes liver inflammation (hepatitis) and nausea. There is no scientific evidence for this assertion.

HOW TO BEGIN NIACIN THERAPY

You might begin with a very low dosage of it, say 50 milligrams. Since we do not want the flushing sensation to startle you, ingest the 50 mgs. at mealtime with a little liquid. The need for "sneaking up" on niacin this way will become apparent.

Note: There are many niacin preparations on the market, available without a prescription. Regular niacin is a crystal that dissolves readily in water. "Modified" or "sustained-release" versions (which usually have an "SR" as part of their name) are often prescribed in the hope that the slower onset of effects will minimize flushing.

If you experience no flushing, no temporary sunburn, continue two or three more times, taking it with a little liquid and food. It is possible that the food itself acts as a buffer, and that the vitamin is being carried along, working like a sustained-release tablet.

You may even receive benefit (though not lowered cholesterol) from this amount, without feeling a thing.

It is rather important, however, to determine whether or not it is being absorbed. In other parts of the world, over the thousands of cases of pellagra studied and treated with niacin, it has been discovered that some people do not absorb the vitamin well.

So to find out, change dosage times to between meals.

Without food to act as a slight buffer, the chances will be increased that you will feel the flushing. Take more water at this time, as dispersal of the nutrient is desirable as the tablet breaks up.

If you still feel no flushing, the possibility exists that you lack another nutrient, pyridoxine hydrochloride: vitamin B-6.

Repeating: You add B-6 if no flushing occurs after several tries. The flushing, you see, is desirable for the primary reason that it proves your capillaries are responding to niacin's antihistamine influence.

Too low histamine, however, provides nothing upon which the niacin can work to open and enlarge your bloodstream. Vitamin B-6 will assist your making sufficient histamine to trigger the needed reaction.

Use between 100 and 200 milligrams of this vitamin with one or two meals a day.

If B-6 fails to produce the temporary sunburn, you should increase the niacin gradually, until flushing does occur. Move to 100 mgs. with meals or between meals.

Many people consume 500 mgs. at a time--this is half a gram. Therapeutic dosages begin at around 1 gram (1,000 mgs.) daily, and increase up to 3 grams (3,000 mgs.) spread out through the day.

Warning: Such large amounts should not be considered without professional advice. The Harvard Heart Letter advises that niacin therapy should be started at a low dose--such as 100 mg three times per day. This amount can be gradually raised to a full dose over three or four months. The suggested level to bring your intake to is one, two or three grams daily, spreading out multiple doses as you wish.

A point will be reached where you know the reaction is taking place. This is benign, harmless and extremely beneficial. What you are experiencing in this nutritive "sunburn" (which lasts from thirty minutes to two hours) is your own fresh blood surging like culverts of released flood water into microscopic capillaries which have been closed for--who knows how long?

The sensation is not unlike when your arm or leg has "gone to sleep," and is beginning to wake up. In both cases, circulation has been stanched and then reopened.

Capillaries which have been damaged (often by real sunburn) react to niacin. But tissues which have not been narrowed and are not refusing blood flow, remain open, and no flushing occurs there, none necessary.

In the gym, you may see bodybuilders turn pink in all the areas where real sunburns in years past have caused microscopic damage to millions of minute blood vessels. The color is deepest around shoulders, across the face, chest and calves. Where swimsuits have protected the body, there may be no niacin flush, and the skin appears normal.

A truck driver whose arm rests on the left-hand windowsill of his vehicle will have more flushing on that arm, because the blood vessels in the skin have suffered more damage from the sun than the protected arm.

HOW NIACIN HELPS MORE THAN THE HEART

What do these unusual symptoms tell us? They tell us that niacin is at work, and it mechanically seeks out areas where blood flow is insufficient.

The niacin reaction depends upon the fact that red blood cells are virtually the exact same diameter as normal capillaries. Free-flowing blood courses along those tiny blood vessels, but, as you can imagine, they inch along single file.

We have already discussed "sludged" blood-- how sticky blood piles up around the entrance to a narrow cell. With red cells barely clearing floor and ceiling as they move through the passage, it should be very clear (to anyone who has tried to move furniture) that if the doorway isn't wide enough, you won't get through.

That is the condition down in the tiniest capillaries of your body. Red cells will not pass through, not only because of sludged blood, but because of roughness, injury or any kind of debris, collections of dead cells and, worst of all, the contraction of the blood vessels themselves.

Fear may cause contraction of the entire arterial system. Cold will do the same. A blow, pressure upon the skin, cigarette smoke, the smoke itself, toxins, drugs--virtually anything that stresses the body, the mind, the emotions, will cause the capillaries throughout the body to shrink, sometimes chemically pulled tight; but also as if pulling away, withdrawing, literally shrinking away. Dehydration shrinks tissues, and all scar tissue shrinks as it heals imperfectly, building defenses against further injury; but also lacking sufficient vitamins A, C and E and other nutrients for perfect repair.

Sometimes the injuries themselves deform tissues so that healing cannot properly take place. No single thing takes place alone, but whatever operates one place, operates in millions of places. For we are composed of billions of cells, and a "condition" impinges upon as many.

When the damage of free-radicals causes damage to cells, when ultraviolet light changes structure, also causing free-radical aging; when worry reduces enzymes; when toxins in the body cannot be carried away, wrong structures get built out of necessity. All these forces clog up blood vessels. We are scarcely aware of any of it.

Suppose you had a bad sunburn once, but have long forgotten it. Yet, on the microscopic level, there will be scars. Free-radical damage, day after day, deposits pigments in skin, building liver spots--and these are equalled by as much pigment in the brain, interfering with neural circuits of thought, comprehension, reaction, memory.

Thus, niacin, in flooding into dried-out "river beds," flows like a flash flood, sweeping the debris of drought, wind, summer and earthquake aside, pushing it through, pulling it back, washing it along, until the artery is clean, and free-flowing once again.

Only from truly grasping this flushing action can we begin to tie together the wide range of disorders which yield to niacin: cholesterol, high blood pressure, MÇniäre's syndrome (dizziness which may be caused or aggravated by circulatory starvation of the middle ear) and pellagra. Dozens of disorders, large and small, yield simply because almost everything is going to change when blood starts flowing once again through all the old, dried-out pipes, and life and moisture, all your nutrition, begin to enrich your debilitated serum once again.

GO WITH THE 'FLUSH'

Because of this radical sweeping through the flesh, your own bloodstream clearing the way for oxygen, the niacin effect is actually very much like free exercise. (We have already mentioned how bodybuilding athletes use niacin to simulate the "pump.")

Because of this kinship to actual exercise, your heart may beat a little faster, and this is a grand time to drink more good water. Thin down your blood quickly, to ease the flow, thin the blood further, so that more capillaries can be reached.

Rather than fighting the sensation, or hating the slight tingle of this temporary sunburn, you should do all in your power to enhance its effect. Make a point of breathing deeply, so that those red cells can bring in more supplies, more oxygen and get the job done right.

It disturbs us when we hear (as we often do) that women shrink from the niacin effect, or refuse to use niacin because they hate the itch, or don't like the palpitations. It is understandable, of course, because, with no knowledge whatever of what really is going on during that odd flushing sensation, they fall back on their usual inclinations.

But niacin, by flushing our debris, opening capillaries by the million, reclaiming hundreds, thousands of lost bloodstream miles, simply makes more interior space for the blood itself. Capillaries, arteries and veins are the total area allowed. There can be no more room or space or territory in your body for your blood than in your native, original system.

When niacin begins to restore that primal, gigantic area--to your arterial and venous system--the only thing that can interfere in your steady recovery from whatever ails is simply not supplying the blood itself with materials to get the most done.

Such supplies include extra water, already mentioned, and deep breathing, to cheer your red cells on. But day by day, it is vastly important--and should, by now, be getting crystal-clear--just why you must have new and vital enzymes ready, all the nutrients for making repairs on hand. Improper repair leaves you with the same old scar tissues as before.

For this reason, when taking your niacin, knowing you will get a reasonably good flush, dissolve vitamin C or any other desired nutrient into your drinking water. Add the right amount of electrolytes and minerals already "ascorbated" in advance--you can buy these in any health-food store. This "reinforced" water will be an immediate help.

We personally chew vitamin E capsules, breaking them and crunching the E oil with raw apple; and store this away, inside, before we take niacin.

LAST, BUT MAYBE THE BEST

Of those nine steps toward heart health we mentioned in the introduction, we have purposely placed niacin last on the list because it is the most controversial. But it just may be the best; and in its "free exercise" of the entire body, it rivals power-walking.

COMBINE THE 9 STEPS TO HEART HEALTH

Indeed, when you've tried them all out, start the next adventure of combining them. Take your niacin, get a good, wholesome "burn" going and then take your leisurely morning stroll. Years will fall away, because this is very much how your body used to feel when it was younger, had more vigor and more blood flowed through those scarred, closed- down blood vessels.

Perhaps you will understand why Dr. Alexis Carrel, that Nobel Prize-winning researcher, claimed we are as old as our serum.

In terms of all that you have discovered herein, think about that. How old is your blood serum? You can feed it, you can moisten it, you can use brans and fiber to clean it and, in fact, what can't you provide?

The unknowns--but that is precisely what a large part of this effort has been about. Why take poor, ruined foods, cooked to death, in all the wrong amounts, when

you can find those unknowns in so many natural foods--
and for so little cost?

BEYOND THE 9 STEPS

In outlining our nine steps to heart health, of course
we've touched on many other preventive measures. But
by now you shouldn't be surprised to find out that there
are many other things we haven't touched on-- other
effective alternatives for prevention and treatment of high
cholesterol and high blood pressure. Some of them are a
little offbeat perhaps, others are downright astonishing,
but we think all are worth investigating. So please read
on.

Notes:

_____

_____

_____

_____

_____

_____

_____

_____

XIII: CAN BAD THINGS BE GOOD FOR YOU?

DON'T NEGLECT YOUR VICES

The actor Hal Holbrook, in his one-man show, "Mark Twain Tonight," retells one of the great American writer's favorite curmudgeonly stories. It seems a man in sinking health went to see his doctor and was told to give up smoking.

"But I don't smoke," protested the man.

"Give up drink then."

"I don't drink either," came the reply.

"What bad habits do you have?" the doctor asked.

"None," the patient said proudly.

"Then you're beyond help," was the doctor's gloomy verdict. "You've neglected your vices. You're like a sinking ship with no ballast to throw overboard."

No, we're not advocating vice here, just moderation. Smoking is verboten, if you want a long and productive life. But we're not fanatics about secondhand smoke or those who enjoy an occasional cigar of pipe.

And some "vices," like alcohol in moderation, can actually be good for you, as we will document. And others, like coffee (also in moderation), appear to be quite harmless, if not exactly benign. So take Twain's advice. You'll live just as long and enjoy the living more en route.

ALCOHOL AND YOUR HEART

Many people were tempted to pop some corks a few years back, when the first reports were published that alcohol might offer health benefits--including a lessening risk for heart disease.

The debate has swung back and forth in recent years, but finally a consensus is emerging--at least as concerns moderate alcohol intake.

Heavy alcohol use is definitely harmful to the liver, heart and other organs. In fact, heavy alcohol intake increases risk of death from all causes, including liver disease; cancers of certain organs; and some types of cardiovascular disease such as heart failure, sudden death due to heart-rhythm abnormalities and hemorrhagic (bleeding) strokes.

But moderate alcohol consumption seems to reduce the risk of coronary artery disease. Light-to-moderate drinkers tend to have lower total mortality rates than both heavy drinkers and nondrinkers. The lower death rate at light- to-moderate levels appears to be largely due to a reduction in coronary artery disease mortality.

Lower rates of coronary artery disease show up at levels as low as three drinks per week. (In these clinical trials, a drink is defined as 12 ounces of beer, 5 ounces of wine, or 1.5 ounces of distilled spirits, all of which contain approximately the same amounts of alcohol.)

New And Natural Ways To Your Lower Blood Pressure, Cholesterol And Stress

The most popular explanation is that alcohol raises high-density-lipoprotein (HDL) cholesterol--the "good" cholesterol associated with a reduced risk of heart attack. As we've discussed, HDL cholesterol is produced primarily in the liver and intestines and is released into the bloodstream. HDL binds with cholesterol and brings it back to the liver for elimination or reprocessing, thereby lowering total cholesterol levels in body tissues.

Another way in which alcohol might lower heart-attack rates, research suggests, is by altering the body's blood-clotting system. Clot formation is an important step in the development of a heart attack. When fats build up on the artery wall, the resulting plaque can rupture, causing a clot to form at the site and to block blood flow completely. This complete blockage of blood flow is the final cause of most heart attacks.

Does it matter what one drinks? Some experts have thought that red wine might reduce the risk of heart disease better than other alcoholic beverages.

This theory has been offered as a possible explanation for the so-called "French Paradox"--the lower-than-expected coronary-artery disease mortality rates in France as well as other Mediterranean countries, despite a relatively high incidence of smoking and high-fat diets. (See more on French Paradox below.)

The theorists note that antioxidants in red wine might enhance its ability to reduce the risk of cardiovascular disease. In addition, red wine may be more effective than white wine at reducing platelet stickiness. Despite these potential advantages for red wine, no clear advantage has been demonstrated yet for any one type of alcoholic beverage. Wine, beer, distilled spirits--all appear to be associated with a lowered risk of coronary artery disease.

A recent study of differences in heart-disease rates in various European countries suggests the level of alcohol content in wine--rather than the total volume or type of wine--was the best predictor of the reduction in risk of death from coronary artery disease. Thus, the major beneficial component of alcoholic beverages may be alcohol itself, not some other ingredient.

CABERNET OR CHARDONNAY?

Scientists have done several followup studies, trying to answer the question, "Which wine is better for the heart, red or white?" Unfortunately, they've come up with differing answers.

In one French test, rats were given white wine, red wine or 6 percent ethanol. At first, all three groups of rodents showed about a 70 percent reduction in the clumping of blood platelets. But when deprived of alcohol for 18 hours, the platelet-clotting response increased 46 percent in the white wine group and 124 percent in the ethanol group. The red wine-drinking rats, however, showed a desirable 59 percent drop in clotting response.

Score one for Cabernet (or Beaujolais or Merlot, or whatever red pleases you).

But the opposite results were reached in a study by researchers at the Kenneth L. Jordan Heart Foundation and Research Center in Montclair, New Jersey. In this trial, twenty men and women with high cholesterol counts drank 180 milliliters of either red or white wine every day for a month, then switched to the other type for another month. (They were allowed to eat whatever they wanted.) Neither group showed any significant changes in total or HDL cholesterol, but LDL cholesterol dropped in the white wine group from 167 to 155 ml/dl. (Both groups showed a decreased blood-clotting response.)

A point for white wine. All even?

That's what researchers at the Kaiser Permanente Medical Care Program in Oakland, California, concluded, after analyzing both red- and white-wine drinkers. Both groups reduced risks of coronary heart disease.

Conclusion: You can find medical experts on both sides of the controversy, while other experts maintain there's no difference. The only scientific consensus? Either one can help lower the risk of developing coronary heart disease.

THE FRENCH PARADOX

Sales of red wine in America rose dramatically soon after the 1991 "60 Minutes" report on the so-called French Paradox, which pointed out the lower rates of heart disease among the French--even though they have a far fattier diet than most Americans--and attributed it to regular consumption of red wine.

On the same day of the "60 Minutes" broadcast in 1991, a front-page story in the New York Times reported on a 10-year French epidemiological study of the dietary effects of duck and goose fat, in the form of foie gras and otherwise. The surprising result of the study, according to Dr. Serge Renaud, director of research at the French National Institute of Health and Medical Research in Lyon, was the discovery that these dangerous-sounding substances might actually be beneficial to the human circulatory system--might actually help clear arteries rather than clogging them. "Goose and duck fat," Renaud explained, "is closer in chemical composition to olive oil than it is to butter or lard."

Today the best nutritionists in the world recognize that the two countries with the lowest rate of heart disease are Japan and France. In France, the region where there is the least heart disease is the Southwest--and that is where they eat the most fat.

And there's more. Japan and France seem to be the two countries with the most old people. So nutritionists around the world are asking themselves how one can live so long, and with so little heart disease, on French cuisine with their emphasis on fats and butter.

* Heavy Lunches, Light Dinners? Perhaps one factor contributing to the paradox is the way of eating. In France they eat a small breakfast and a big lunch-- a lunch much bigger than dinner. (This is especially true in the countryside.)

This, of course, is the reverse of the American eating pattern. We eat a big breakfast, practically skip lunch, and then have the biggest meal for dinner. But nutritionists agree that it is not a good to eat a lot in the evening.

An interesting corroboration appears in Dr. Deepak Chopra's book, "Perfect Weight." According to Chopra, Ayurveda (discussed in Chapter 13), the ancient Indian system of natural medicine, the body's "digestive fire" burns strongest at midday. Which means that digestion is most active at that time, so the body is able to convert food into energy more efficiently after lunch.

So Dr. Chopra also recommends making lunch the largest meal. Try it--and see if it doesn't improve your metabolism!

A TOAST TO WOMANKIND

Several pioneering studies on the coronary benefits of light drinking were conducted among men. So Harvard researchers studied the relationship between alcohol consumption and the risk of dying among 85,709 women participating in the Nurses' Health Study (which followed 121,700 female registered nurses who enrolled in the investigation in 1976).

Most women reported less than one drink a day. The overall risk of death from all causes among light drinkers was about 14% lower than the risk for women who drank not at all and for those who drank 30 or more grams of alcohol per day. Most of this difference reflected a substantial decrease in heart- attack risk.

Women with one or more risk factors for heart disease appeared even more likely than others to benefit from light drinking. These risk factors include cigarette smoking, high blood pressure, high blood-cholesterol levels, obesity, a family history of heart disease and a history of diabetes. In general, women who had a couple of drinks were less likely to die from heart disease or other causes than the teetotalers.

CAUTION: TRIGLYCERIDES AND ALCOHOL

While studies have shown that a drink or two a day can help raise HDL cholesterol, alcohol can actually raise triglycerides by lowering the concentration of an enzyme used to break them down. "Even having a glass of wine with dinner every night can substantially raise triglycerides in people who are overweight or who have hereditary triglyceride problems," says Thomas Bersot, M.D., associate professor of medicine at the University of California, San Francisco.

SAY YES TO SEX

Heart patients and their partners often fear that sex will trigger a heart attack. But, according to findings from a Harvard Medical School test, these are groundless fears. Most of the 11 million Americans with heart disease can relax and enjoy sex whenever they want.

The study followed 1,774 patients who had suffered heart attacks, including 858 who were sexually active in the year before. Among them, 27 reported sexual activity in the two hours preceding the attacks. The study indicates that the actual risk of a heart attack is quite low--about as risky per episode as getting angry or waking up in the morning. In fact, heavy exertion can be three times riskier than any of those activities.

GOOD NEWS FOR SMOKERS?

If you've been paying attention so far, you know that there's nothing good to be said about cigarette smoking. It's almost a guaranteed ticket to cardiac disease.

Despite that, there is a bit of good news for cigarette smokers.

A pioneering medical study (published in the American Heart Association journal, Circulation, July, 1996) found that injections of vitamin C given to smokers can reverse one of the most harmful cardiovascular effects of smoking.

The vitamin works because of its antioxidant function, said Dr. Thomas Munzel of the University of Freiburg in Germany, one of the study's authors.

Cigarette smoke contains powerful oxidants-- chemicals that react like oxygen, which rusts iron and makes peeled apples turn brown. High concentrations of vitamin C or vitamin E neutralize oxidants.

The study suggests that in people, oxidants damage the endothelium, a layer of cells that helps arteries narrow and widen. When the endothelium is damaged, plaque forms more easily in the arteries, making people more prone to strokes and heart attacks.

Researchers gave injections of a chemical that stimulates the endothelial cells to 10 nonsmokers and 10 longtime smokers. This caused the nonsmokers' arteries to widen, but it had a much weaker effect on the smokers.

The researchers then injected vitamin C directly

into their bloodstreams and tried the first chemical again. The nonsmokers' arteries widened as they had before, but now the smokers' arteries responded equally well.

The process "almost completely reverses endothelial dy- sfunction in chronic smokers," the researchers said. Other scientists cautioned that this does not definitively prove that vitamin C neutralizes the effect of smoking on heart disease.

Another study in which smokers were given vitamin C pills over eight years found no effect on their rate of heart disease, said Eric Rimm, an assistant professor of epidemiology at the Harvard School of Public Health.

"I think vitamin C among smokers is very important," Rimm said. The new study "does suggest that vitamin C has an acute effect of stopping vascular dysfunction.

But he cautioned: "It's too early to make the leap that vit min C will protect smokers from heart disease."

(AND SOME NEW BAD NEWS...)

New medical research shows how a "molecular glue" may stick to smokers' arteries, raising their risk of heart disease.

Heart disease accounts for nearly half of the 419,000 smoking-related deaths in the United States each year. The research, presented to the Molecular Medicine Society, gave some insight into the cause.

Anthony Cerami, a scientist at the Picower Institute in Manhasset, New York, said a blood test found high levels of "advanced glycation end products"

(AGEs) in smokers' blood. AGEs are found in cigarette smoke and are formed when tobacco leaves are dried.

Once in the bloodstream, they form a "molecular glue" that sticks to the arterial walls, constricting circulation and causing hardening of the arteries. That in turn creates a risk for heart attack or stroke.

"This study is significant because it offers new evidence that in the process of drying tobacco leaves, compounds are produced which are carried in the smoke to the lungs where they react in the body and induce vascular disease," said Cerami.

He said a blood test could help doctors better assess the health risks of their patients who smoke.

The study found higher AGE levels in 23 smokers than it did in 13 people in a control group. Similar results were found in rats exposed to smoke for 22 months.

Cerami is best known for developing a glucose test for diabetics who are at risk of a similar kind of vascular disease.

COFFEE VS. CHOLESTEROL: WHAT'S THE SCORE?

Back in the early '60s the first medical studies came out linking coffee-drinking to higher cholesterol. One study of 2,000 men over a seven-year period found that those who developed coronary disease drank five cups of coffee or more per day.

This was given more weight when scientists found that even a single cup of coffee causes a prompt rise in blood fats and cholesterol.

Decaffeinated brews were offered as one possible way out for coffee drinkers, since they seem not to have these cholesterol-raising effects.

But the controversy has been going on and on, with more reports, more studies, and a lot of scientific disagreement. Some found problems even with decaf. Others investigated the different kinds of beans--arabica vs. robusta.

The preponderance of evidence, however, points not to coffee itself as the problem, not what kind of beans. Not "caff" versus "decaf," but the way the coffee is prepared--boiled or filtered. One study in the Netherlands found that those drinking unfiltered, boiled coffee experienced an average increase in total and LDL cholesterol of 16 milligrams. While those drinking filtered coffee had no cholesterol rise at all.

What caused the dramatic difference? Apparently, according to careful followup research, it's fatty substances in coffee--substances which are effectively trapped in the filters--that hype the cholesterol levels.

("Cafestrol" and "kahweol" are the names of these fats.)

This is welcome news, of course, for those of us who love our coffee (and we plead guilty). We can enjoy our morning brew, so long as we filter it. However, that means we should avoid espresso coffee, French press coffee, Turkish coffee, Scandinavian boiled coffee, and other gourmet preparations that don't use a filter.

HOW MUCH IS TOO MUCH?

So long as we follow these simple filtration guidelines, and drink in "moderation" (no more than five cups per day, three being even better), we are running no real health risk, according to most scientific opinion.

Drinking more than three cups per day results in elevated blood lipids, and above five cups daily is associated with heart attacks.

Since this is not true of tea or cola drinks, it seems that caffeine is not the culprit. Caffeine does seem to cause a slight rise in blood pressure, but this seems to be short-term. As for the cream some of us like in our coffee, that's a separate issue, which we've already discussed under the issue of dietary fats.

ADDITIONAL COMMENTS ON COFFEE

There are other health reasons for kicking the caffeine habit, however. And if you want to verify that it is an addiction, try going "cold turkey"--and you may experience classic withdrawal symptoms-- i.e, nausea, headache, even fatigue.

Fatigue? Yes, oddly enough, too much caffeine can cause an afternoon letdown. Caffeine gives us its jolt by stimulating the liver to release stored sugar. But this is a short-term effect, and as it wears thin, you may experience fatigue.

Other common and undesirable effects of too much caffeine consumption include irritability, insomnia and jittery nerves.

Worse than all of these, however, may be caffeine's "sapping" effect on vitamins and minerals. In fact, much of the caffeine-fatigue syndrome is due to the loss of these nutrients, particularly B-vitamins.

Note: Kicking the coffee habit does not necessarily get you off caffeine. As mentioned previously, the stimulant is present is soft drinks, painkillers, diet pills and drugstore stimulants.

Final footnote: There was once speculation that caffeine could contribute to birth defects. More recent studies, however, have shown that moderate amounts of coffee (1 to 2 cups daily) are quite safe for pregnant women.

PASS THE TEA

Dietitians at one time considered tea not on the recommended list due to its caffeine content. But more recent research shows that tea has only half the caffeine of coffee. And, according to studies at the University of Scranton in Pennsylvania, both black and green tea contain antioxidants that help keep LDL cholesterol from clogging arteries. There had been previous studies of Asian drinkers of green and oolong teas, which indicated that those were superior in health benefits. But the Scranton studies indicate that black teas may have just as many benefits.

Teas both black and green contain a class of beneficial phytochemicals called polyphenols. A series of tests in China, the Netherlands and the U.S. show that polyphenols in tea help to reduce the risk of several diseases that lead to premature aging.

Another survey published in 1995 in the British Medical Journal showed that Japanese men who

drank the most tea had 5.5 percent lower total cholesterol, 12 percent less triglyceride and 3 percent higher
HDLs than those who drank no tea.

The substances in tea that possess the antioxidant effect are flavonoids. Flavonoids also dilate coronary blood vessels, lower blood lipids and stabilize
arterial walls. They also seem to act to inhibit an
enzyme, ACE, which helps create high blood pressure.
In fact, they function similar to the drug captopril, commonly given to combat high blood pressure.

A study in the Netherlands found that men who
consumed the most flavonoids had less than a third
the number of fatal heart attacks compared with those
who consumed the fewest. Though flavonoids are present in fruits and vegetables, those in the Dutch study
came mostly from tea.

Another source of dietary flavonoids: red wine
and grape juice.

HEALTH CLAIMS FOR 'PENTA' TEA

Another tea for which some extravagant (and so
far unverified) health claims have been made is Penta
Tea. Penta's Chinese name is Jaogulan, or JGL, and it
has been used in China as a vegetable and a tea for
many centuries. It's a herb that belongs to the cucumber family.

Its distributors claims that pharmacological
experiments and clinical studies conducted in China
show that jaogulan saponins has a beneficial effect on
high blood fats, atherosclerosis, thrombosis and senility. They also believe that penta tea or concentrate can
cause your body to behave as if your liver were fit, that
regular consumption of penta can dramatically lower

overall serum cholesterol levels and raise HDL or good cholesterol levels.

For information, e-mail for the booklet, "A Gem from the Orient," call (800) 251-8840 or (207) 652-2206, or write to Natural Health, PO Box 274, New Vineyard, ME 04956-0274.

DON'T FORGET THE MAYO

Surprising evidence is building that reasonable amounts of mayonnaise and salad dressing--shunned by many because they are so high in fat--can be an important part of a heart-healthy diet because they are good sources of vitamin E.

MAKING THE BEST OF FAST FOODS

It's almost impossible for many of us to pass up an occasional fast-food meal. Convenience is an important factor for almost everybody. Meals made in advance or frozen fulfill a need, and so do take-outs and drive-throughs. Busy folks can grab a drive-through lunch or a take-home dinner for the family, an easy and fairly inexpensive alternative to home cooking or dining out at more expensive restaurants.

Of course, many fast-food items are high in calories, fats, cholesterol and sodium. A single meal can easily exceed the recommended values for an entire day. But with a little care, fast foods can be a part of a healthy food chain.

Avoid combining the jumbo cheeseburgers (1,000 calories, 80 grams of fat, 200 mg of cholesterol, 1200 mg of sodium) with jumbo fries (400 calories, 20 grams of fat, 200 mg sodium).

Most fast-food franchises offer salads, for instance, providing salad dressings on the side--and you can request low-fat or fat-free dressing. Otherwise, a salad with chicken (200 calories, 9 grams of fat) can be a fattening meal if you pour on 300 calories of high-fat dressing.

Okay, you like fries and an occasional burger. It's not the best way to get your beef, but get the small order, the smaller burger. You'll get the same taste sensation, but won't feel bloat- ed and heavy afterward.

And some fast-food menus now include chicken and turkey dishes, including grilled sandwiches and fajitas, salads and fresh vegetables. And some Mexican take-outs offer a "light" menu with 50 percent less fat.

Suggested "best bet" fast-food lunches:

McDonald's: Chef salad and vanilla shake. 460 calories, 28 grams protein, 10 grams fat, 50 percent calcium, 8 percent iron.

Burger King: Broiled chicken salad, vegetable sticks, Weight Watchers creamy ranch dressing and frozen yogurt. 360 calories, 21 grams protein, 9 grams fat, 18 percent calcium, 14 percent iron.

Hardee's: Ham sub, side salad with fat-free dressing. 390 calories, 27 grams protein, 7 grams fat, 27 percent calcium, 27 percent iron.

Wendy's: Grilled chicken sandwich, 8 ounces 2 percent milk, vegetable salad with four tablespoons picante sauce. 470 calories, 32 grams protein, 11 grams fat, 40 percent calcium, 20 percent iron.

Roy Rogers: Roast beef sandwich with plenty of "Fixin's" (lettuce, tomatoes, pickles, onions, mustard), and a 7-ounce orange juice. 416 calories, 27 grams protein, 10 grams fat, 9 percent calcium, 23 percent iron.

BEATING THE SNACK ATTACK

Do you have a tendency to stop off at the dough-nut shop on the way to work? You can make the stop but order a bagel instead of a cruller.

Drinking too much coffee, tea, and cola out of habit? Take a water bottle and keep it keep handy.

Are you a habitual muncher? Take along a Ziploc bag full of baby carrots, celery sticks, cauliflower and broccoli florets, zucchini and yellow squash slices, cucumber chunks, radishes and cherry tomatoes. You'll not only have plenty to chomp, but will be getting lots of fiber, anti-oxidant vitamins and phytochemicals to reduce your risks of cancer and heart disease.

If you like mushy foods, reach for a ripe banana or a carton of fat-free yogurt instead of a doughnut or candy bar.

Some other good emergency snackers:

* 3-ounce pop-top can of tuna.

* Hunt's Snack Pack light vanilla pudding.

* DelMonte Fruit Snax orchard mix package.

* Individually wrapped bread sticks.

* 8-ounce box of orange juice.

* 1-ounce package of salted peanuts.

NUTRITIONAL CONTENT OF FAST FOODS

Fast Foods

	Calories (gm)	Fat (mg)	Chol. (mg)	Sodium Fat	% Fat
ARBY'S					
Junior Roast Beef	218	9	20	345	37
Regular Roast Beef	353	15	39	588	39
Giant Roast Beef	531	23	65	908	39
Philly Beef'N Swiss	460	28	107	1300	55
King Roast Beef	467	19	49	766	37
Super Roast Beef	501	22	40	798	40
Beef'N Cheddar	455	27	63	955	53
Bac'N Cheddar Deluxe	526	37	83	1672	63
Chicken Breast Sandwich	509	29	83	1082	51
Turkey Deluxe	375	17	39	1047	41
Hot Ham'N Cheese	292	14	45	1350	43
Fish Fillet Sandwich	580	32	70	928	50
Potato Cakes	.201	13	13	397	58
BURGER KING					
Whopper Sandwich	628	36	90	880	52
w/cheese	711	43	113	1164	54
Bacon Double Cheesebur	510	31	104	728	55
Whopper Junior Sandwich	322	17	41	486	48
w/cheese	364	20	52	628	49
Hamburger	275	12	37	509	39
Cheeseburger	317	15	48	651	43
Ham & Cheese Sandwich	471	23	70	1534	44

New And Natural Ways To Your Lower Blood Pressure, Cholesterol And Stress

Chicken Sandwich	688	40	82	1423	52
Chicken Tenders (6 pcs.)	204	10	47	636	44
Whaler Fish Sandwich	488	27	77	592	50
Garden Salad	110	6	10	170	49
Side Salad	20	0	0	10	0
Chef Salad	180	11	120	610	55
Chunky Chicken Salad	140	4	50	440	26
Breakfast Croissan'wich	304	19	243	637	56
w/bacon	355	24	248	762	61
w/sausage	538	41	293	1042	69
w/ham	335	20	262	987	54
Bagel, Egg & Cheese					
w/bacon	438	19	273	905	39
w/ham	418	15	286	1130	32
w/sausage	621	36	317	1185	52
Scrambled Egg Platter	468	30	370	808	58
w/sausage	700	52	420	1213	67
w/bacon	536	58	378	975	97
French Toast Sticks	499	29	74	498	52
Great Danish	500	36	6	288	65
Cookies & Cream Spooner	270	10	N.A.	210	33
CHURCH'S FRIED CHICKEN					
Breast	278	17	N.A.	560	55
Wing Breast	303	20	N.A.	583	59
Thigh	306	22	N.A.	448	65
Leg	147	9	N.A.	286	55
Corn-on-the-Cob, buttered	237	9	N.A.	20	34

New And Natural Ways To Your Lower Blood Pressure, Cholesterol And Stress

DAIRY QUEEN

Single Hamburger	360	16	45	630	40
w/cheese	410	20	50	790	44
Double Hamburger	530	28	85	660	48
w/cheese	650	37	95	980	51
Chicken Sandwich	640	41	75	870	58
Fish Sandwich	400	17	50	875	38
w/cheese	440	21	60	1035	43
Hot Dog	280	16	45	830	51
w/chili	320	20	55	985	56
w/cheese	330	21	55	990	57
Super Hot Dog	520	27	80	1365	47
w/chili	570	32	100	1595	51
w/cheese	580	34	100	1605	53
DQ Dip Cone, small	190	9	10	55	42
regular	340	16	20	100	42
large	510	24	30	145	42
DQ Banana Split	540	11	30	150	18
Hot Fudge Brownie Delight	600	25	20	225	38

JACK IN THE BOX

Hamburger	267	11	26	556	37
Cheeseburger	315	14	41	746	40
Double Cheeseburger	467	27	72	842	52
Jumbo Jack	584	34	73	733	52
Jumbo Jack w/cheese	677	40	102	1090	53
Bacon Cheeseburger	705	39	85	1127	50
Swiss & Bacon Burger	678	47	92	1458	62
Ultimate Cheeseburger	942	69	127	1176	66

New And Natural Ways To Your Lower Blood Pressure, Cholesterol And Stress

Chicken Supreme	575	36	62	1525	56
Grilled Chicken Sandwich	447	19	N.A.	845	38
Chicken Strips (6 pcs.)	523	20	103	1122	34
Fish Supreme	554	32	66	1047	52
Shrimp (10 pcs.)	270	16	84	669	53
Beef Fajita Pita	333	14	45	635	38
Chicken Fajita Pita	292	8	34	703	25
Club Pita w/o sauce	277	8	43	431	26
Hot Club Supreme	524	28	82	1467	48
Taco	191	11	21	406	51
Super Taco	288	17	37	765	53
Guacamole	55	5	0	130	81
Egg Rolls (3 pcs.)	405	19	30	903	42
Chef Salad	325	18	142	900	50
Mexican Chicken Salad	443	21	104	1530	43
Taco Salad	641	38	91	1670	53
Side Salad	51	3	4	84	53
Supreme Crescent	547	40	178	1053	66
Sausage Crescent	584	43	187	1012	66
Canadian Crescent	452	31	226	851	62
Breakfast Jack	307	13	203	871	38
Egg Platter	662	40	354	1188	54
Hash Browns	116	7	3	211	54
Pancake Platter	612	22	99	888	32
Cheesecake	309	18	63	208	52

KENTUCKY FRIED CHICKEN

Original Recipe Chicken

Wing	118	12	67	387	92

New And Natural Ways To Your Lower Blood Pressure, Cholesterol And Stress

Side Breast	276	17	96	654	55
Center Breast	257	14	93	532	49
Drumstick	147	9	81	269	55
Thigh	278	19	122	517	62
Extra Crispy Chicken					
Wing	218	16	63	437	66
Side Breast	354	24	66	797	61
Center Breast	353	21	93	842	54
Drumstick	173	11	65	346	57
Thigh	371	26	121	766	63
Kentucky Nuggets (6 pcs.)	276	17	71	840	55
Mashed Potatoes	59	.5	0	228	8
Mashed Potatoes w/gravy	62	1	0	297	15
Chicken Gravy	59	4	2	398	61
Corn-on-the-Cob	176	3	0	10	15
Cole Slaw	103	6	4	171	52
Potato Salad	141	9	11	396	57
Baked Beans	105	1	0	387	9
Buttermilk Biscuit	269	14	0	521	47
LONG JOHN SILVER'S					
Chicken Planks (4 pcs.)	440	24	60	1280	49
Fish w/batter (2 pcs.)	300	16	60	1020	48
Catfish Fillet (2 pcs.)	400	24	60	700	54
Breaded Shrimp (1 order)	190	10	40	470	47
Battered Shrimp (6 pcs.)	240	18	60	720	68
Breaded Clams	240	12	<5	410	45
Crispy Breaded Fish Sandwich	600	28	30	1220	42
Clam Chowder w/cod (7 oz.)	140	6	20	590	39

New And Natural Ways To Your Lower Blood Pressure, Cholesterol And Stress

Gumbo (7 oz.)	120	8	25	740	60
Seafood Salad w/2 crackers	270	7	90	660	23
Ocean Chef Salad w/2 crackers	250	9	80	1340	32
Cole Slaw	140	6	15	260	39
Mixed Vegetables	60	2	0	330	30
Corn-on-the-Cob, buttered	270	14	<5	95	47
Hushpuppies (3 pcs.)	210	6	<5	75	26
Pecan Pie (1 slice)	530	25	70	470	42
Lemon Meringue Pie (1 slice)	260	7	<5	270	24
McDONALD'S					
Hamburger	263	11	29	506	38
Cheeseburger	318	16	41	743	45
Quarter Pounder	427	24	81	718	51
w/cheese	525	32	107	1220	55
Big Mac	570	35	83	979	55
McD.LT.	680	44	101	1030	58
Chicken McNuggets (6 pcs.)	323	21	73	512	59
Filet-O-Fish	435	26	45	799	54
Chef Salad	226	13	125	850	52
Shrimp Salad	99	3	187	570	27
Garden Salad	91	6	110	100	59
Chicken Salad Oriental	146	4	92	270	25
Side Salad	48	3	42	45	56
Egg McMuffin	340	16	259	885	42
Sausage McMuffin	427	26	59	942	55
w/egg	517	33	287	1044	57
Biscuit, Plain	330	18	9	786	49

New And Natural Ways To Your Lower Blood Pressure, Cholesterol And Stress

w/sausage	467	31	48	1147	60
w/sausage & egg	585	40	285	1301	62
w/bacon, egg & cheese	483	32	263	1269	60
Scrambled Eggs	180	13	514	205	65
Hot Cakes w/butter & syrup	500	10	47	1070	18
Sausage	210	19	39	423	81
Hash Brown Potatoes	125	7	7	325	50
Engfish Muffin w/butter	186	5	15	310	24
Soft Serve Cone	185	5	24	109	2
Sundae, all flavors	346	10	28	135	26
McDonaldland Cookies	308	11	10	358	32
Chocolate Chip Cookies	342	16	18	313	42

PIZZA HUT

(serving size--2 slices of medium 13-inch. pizza; 4 servings per pizza)

Thin'n Crispy

Standard Cheese	340	11	22	900	29
Superstyle Cheese	410	14	30	1100	31
Standard Pepperoni	370	15	27	1000	36
Superstyle Pepperoni	430	19	34	1200	40
Standard Pork					
w/mushroom	380	14	35	1200	33
Superstyle Pork					
w/mushroom	450	19	40	1400	38
Supreme	400	17	13	1200	38
Super Supreme	520	26	44	1500	45

Thick'n Chewy

Standard Cheese	390	10	18	800	23
Superstyle Cheese	450	14	21	1000	28

New And Natural Ways To Your Lower Blood Pressure, Cholesterol And Stress

Standard Pepperoni	450	16	21	900	32
Superstyle Pepperoni	490	20	24	1200	37
Standard Pork w/mushroom	430	14	21	1000	29
Superstyle Pork w/mushroom	500	18	21	1200	32
Supreme	480	18	24	1000	34
Super Supreme	590	26	38	1400	40
TACO BELL					
Bean Burrito	360	11	14	922	28
Beef Burrito	402	17	59	944	38
Burrito Supreme	422	19	35	952	41
Double Beef Burrito Supreme	465	23	59	1054	45
Tostada	243	11	18	670	41
Enchirito	382	20	56	1260	47
Mexican Pizza	714	48	81	1364	61
Pintos & Cheese	194	9	19	733	42
Nachos	356	19	9	423	48
Nachos Bellgrande	720	41	43	1312	51
Taco	184	11	32	273	54
Taco Bellgrande	351	22	55	470	56
Taco Light	412	29	57	575	63
Soft Taco	229	12	32	516	47
Taco Salad w/salsa	949	62	85	1763	59
Taco Salad w/o shell	525	32	82	1522	55
Fajita Steak Taco	236	11	14	507	42
Chicken Fajita	225	N.A.	N.A.	N.A.	N.A.
Maxi Melt	264	N.A.	N.A.	N.A.	N.A.

New And Natural Ways To Your Lower Blood Pressure, Cholesterol And Stress

Cinnamon Crispas	266	16	2	122	54
Cheesearito	312	13	29	451	38
WENDY'S					
Hamburger	260	9	30	510	31
Cheeseburger	320	15	50	805	42
Single Hamburger	430	22	70	805	46
w/cheese	490	28	95	1100	51
Double Hamburger	640	36	145	910	51
w/cheese	700	42	160	1205	54
Triple Hamburger	850	50	220	1015	50
w/cheese	970	62	250	1605	58
Bacon Cheeseburger	535	31	78	993	52
Philly Swiss Burger	510	24	65	975	42
Bacon Swiss Burger	710	44	90	1390	56
Wendy's Big Classic w/cheese	640	40	100	1310	56
Chicken Breast Fillet	200	10	60	310	45
Chicken Sandwich	430	19	60	705	40
Crispy Chicken Nuggets (6 pcs.)	310	21	50	660	61
Chili	230	9	50	960	35
Hot Stuffed Baked Potatoes Plain (9 oz.)	250	2	0	60	7
Sour Cream/Chives	460	24	15	230	4
Cheese	590	34	22	450	52
Chili & Cheese	510	20	22	610	35
Bacon & Cheese	570	30	22	1180	47
Broccoli & Cheese	500	25	22	430	45
Garden Salad (take-out)	102	5	0	110	44
Chef Salad (take-out)	180	9	120	140	45

New And Natural Ways To Your Lower Blood Pressure, Cholesterol And Stress

Taco Salad	660	37	35	1110	50
Deluxe Three Bean Salad (1/4 cup)	60	0	N.A.	15	0
Red Bliss Potato Salad (1/4 cup)	110	9	N.A.	265	74
Pasta Deli Salad (1/4 cup)	35	0	N.A.	120	0
California Cole Slaw (1/4 cup)	60	6	10	140	90
Turkey Ham (1/4 cup)	50	2	N.A.	N.A.	36
Taco Shell (1)	50	2	N.A.	0	36
Flour Tortilla	110	3	N.A.	220	25
Taco Chips (2 oz.)	260	10	N.A.	20	35
Fettucini (1 cup)	296	7	0	7	21
Rotini (1 cup)	226	5	0	0	1
Pasta Medley (1 cup)	156	5	0	7	29
Alfredo Sauce (1/2 cup)	110	4	N.A.	44	33
Spaghetti Sauce (1/2 cup)	88	0	0	872	0
Cheese Sauce (1/2 cup)	110	4	N.A.	916	33
Frosty (small)	400	14	50	220	32
Pudding, all flavors (1/2 cup)	180	8	0	156	80

* Chol = Cholesterol

N.A. = Not Available

XIV: ALTERNATIVE CURES AND THERAPIES

ALTERATIVE MEDICINE: QUACKERY OR HEALTH RESOURCE?

For most of this century, the western medical establishment has labeled all forms of alternative medicine as pure quackery, and its practitioners as basically purveyors of snake oil.

Finally, that's starting to change. In 1993, the National Institutes of Health (NIH) opened its own Office of Alternative Medicine, researching such unorthodox options as acupuncture, homeopathy, and meditation.

Why the revolutionary about-face? Mainly because of pressure from physicians who had been using these therapies for many years, as well as from patients, who had been demanding them. In fact, in 1992 the New England Journal of Medicine reported that one in three Americans had recently used some form of alternative therapy as part of their medical therapy--a percentage that is on the rise.

More encouraging to those of who believe in the efficacy of these alternative treatments, more than twenty medical schools now offer courses on holistic and alternative medicine studies.

This increased understanding and acceptance of the principles of alternative medicine will have a direct (and beneficial) effect on the millions of Americans suffering or at risk from cardiovascular disease.

As we've shown over and over in the preceding pages, optimum treatment and prevention of heart disease require many options that used to be thought of as outside mainstream medicine: nutrition, exercise, and stress reduction.

But, of course, almost all mainstream cardiologists have incorporated these approaches. While more and more cardiac patients are not satisfied with simply surgically repairing a damaged heart or taking prescription pills to lower blood pressure.

If this expanding attitude toward improved heart health describes you, you might want to consider some additional avenues of alternative medicine.

But, because they are nontraditional, it may help to familiarize yourself with the terminology and the philosophies behind them. Some of them--especially those with roots in Asian religions and medicine--emphasize spiritual aspects that are not usually brought up by Western healers. If any of this makes you uncomfortable--for instance, a prescription for daily meditation--these spiritual options may not be for you.

Also, if you're averse to being massaged or touched by therapists of practitioners, you should avoid any therapies that use massage or other types of physical manipulation. Similarly, an extreme sensitivity to needles would probably rule out acupuncture--unless you can overcome your fears.

And some alternative therapies require very strict dietary changes.

Ayurvedic medicine, a form of yoga, involves detoxifying the body with certain herbs and periods of fasting, as well as eliminating certain foods altogether.

This obviously isn't for everyone.

Caution No. 1: There are no magic bullets or quick fixes in any kind of medicine, including the alternate variety. But patience is a particular requirement of the natural healing process.

Caution No. 2: Yes, there are quacks and snake-oil purveyors out there on the fringes of alternative medicine. So we include guidelines on how to steer a wide path around these charlatans, and on ways to make sure you deal only with licensed and reputable therapists

1. Get a "mainstream" accurate diagnosis. Don't start shopping for alternative therapies or practitioners without first getting certain tests and procedures done. These tests are best administered by a cardiologist at a hospital or clinic. Bring the diagnostic information with you to your first appointment with an alternative practitioner.

2. Study any alternative therapy or therapies that interest you. Read articles and books about the practices, talk to friends and acquaintances with experiences--and don't forget to ask your mainstream physician for his or her opinion.

In fact, try to build a relationship between your mainstream and alternative practitioners. Especially with heart disease, it makes wonderful sense to have the best of both worlds: the lifesaving emergency technology and diagnostics of Western medicine and the holistic, mind-body methods of healing implicit in alternative medicine.

3. Examine credentials carefully. Unlike for mainstream physicians, there are no national licensing requirements for most alternative medicine practitioners. But certification and licensing are done on a state-by-state basis. So check with your local health department for licensing requirements, certification, degrees, and diplomas for holistic practitioners. Or call a national association in the specialty field you are considering.

4. Interview your prospective practitioner. This means before they examine you, you examine them! During this preliminary visit, check out the office for cleanliness and your own feelings of comfort or discomfort. Is the staff cooperative, friendly? Do they respect patient confidentiality?

Specifically ask the practitioner how much experience he or she has had in treating cardiovascular disease.

Ask about the suggested course of treatment and what side effects or adverse reactions are possible from it. How many appointments and how much time will it take before you see improvement in the health of your heart and blood vessels? How much will it likely cost? Find out about payment options and billing procedures.

If you feel uncomfortable in any respect, don't feel obligated to continue.

5. Obtain a second opinion--and this applies to both your mainstream and alternative practitioner. If you have questions or doubts about the course of treatment being prescribed for your cardiovascular disease, find another qualified doctor or practitioner to

evaluate your case.

And never be afraid to change doctors or therapists. While such a decision should not be made lightly, mutual trust and respect are vital to any course of
treatment--especially for cardiovascular disease.

Now, with our brief intro and guidelines out of the
way, here is a short survey of natural therapies currently being used to treat cardiovascular disease:

ACUPUNCTURE AND YOUR HEART

A practitioner of Chinese medicine, after a thorough examination of a patient with heart problems,
might use different diagnostic language. For instance,
he or she might say that the patient's body was in a
state of imbalance, which affected blood pressure and
heart. The practitioner would probably use Chinese
terms, like "qi" (vital life energy), "yin and yang" (internal balance), or "shen" (the spirit that resides in the
heart). (See below for expanded definitions.)

A treatment plan might involve acupuncture to
relax the liver yang, build up the kidney yin and free up
the energy in the heart channel. Typical herbal remedies include Xiao Yao San ("Free and Easy
Wanderer"), which acts to cool out "hot" energy of the
liver, and Hu-po Yang-xin Dan ("Amber Nourishing the
Heart Pill"), which strengthens the heart and stabilizes
the shen.

Also frequently prescribed are qi-gong exercises
that work to build the qi and keep it moving freely
through the body. Acupressure and other massage
techniques might be employed. Finally, standard medical advice is often given, such as to improve his diet,
cut down drinking and lose weight.

Surgery and drugs are not usually a part of Chinese medicine, but followup diagnostic tools, such as specialized x-rays, would certainly be used.

History of Acupuncture: The first major treatise on Chinese medicine dates back thousands of years, outlining an approach to health practiced today by more than one fourth of the world's population. This philosophy of health is based on the view that each individual is part of a larger creation--the universe itself. The flows of bodily fluid and energy are referred to as channels and rivers, and the state of the body as a whole in terms of the natural elements--dryness, heat, cold, dampness, wind.

Chinese philosophy maintains that human beings represent the linking of heaven and earth and thus are a fusion of cosmic and terrestrial forces. When any part of this fusion becomes unbalanced, natural disasters (such as floods or droughts) or human disease may occur. To heal the body, according to this philosophy, is to heal a part of the universe.

Terms defined:

* "Yin/Yang" = Internal Balance

Internal harmony is expressed in Chinese medicine through the principle of yin and yang, in which two opposing forces unite to create everything in the universe. Yin is associated with cold, dark, and wet, while yang is bright, warm and dry. Yin is quiet, static, inactive. Yang is dynamic, active and expansive.

Chinese medicine views parts of the body as having more yin or more yang qualities. Indeed, every organ is seen to be more yin or yang. "Yin" organs are the heart, spleen, lungs, kidney, and liver. The "yang" organs are the small intestine, stomach, large intestine and bladder. The organs work in mutual support and balance to maintain balance within the organism. When yin/yang becomes upset, symptoms that we recognize as disease and ill health can occur.

* "Qi" = Life Force

Chinese medicine holds that health is maintained when energy, known as "qi" (pronounced "chee") flows freely through the body. "Qi" is the energy essential for life, and health is determined by a sufficient, balanced and uninterrupted flow of qi.

If qi becomes blocked along one of your "meridians" (the paths through which it flows), the organ meant to be nourished by this energy will not receive enough life force to perform its functions. By locating the blockage and releasing it, Chinese therapists attempt to restore energy flow.

Example: Angina, a major symptom of heart disease, is often felt in the arm, along the heart meridian.

WHAT HAPPENS WHEN YOU VISIT AN ACUPUNCTURIST

Practitioners of Chinese medicine attempt to treat disease by restoring yin/yang and a healthy qi flow to the body. Americans used to Western medicine may be surprised by the kind of examination they receive from a practitioner of Chinese medicine. The emphasis will probably be on discussing any symptoms that prompted your visit, as well as aspects of your life and lifestyle that may shed light on your health.

The doctor may ask how you react to heat and cold, dampness and dryness, seasonal variations and day-to-night changes in mood and feelings of well-being. Other questions may concern bowel movements, menstruation and eating and drinking habits. Your answers will provide the doctor an idea of what part of your system is out of balance and what kind of treatment you may need to restore internal harmony.

Acupuncturists also places a great deal on your pulse. In fact, he or she will feel twelve different pulses, six on each side. The doctor may also spend time looking at your tongue--specifically its coating, color and shape. Again, this is an attempt to locate where in your body qi has been disrupted.

Chinese practitioners may also press on the stomach to feel for tenderness, warm or cool areas, and a pulse in the belly button.

Finally, your Chinese doctor will feel along the "meridians" for signs of tenderness, temperature changes and other irregularities. The belief in Chinese medicine is that heart disease can often be traced to a problem in the liver meridian. In fact, the liver is called "the mother of the heart." (Chinese doctors hold that heart problems may also trace to problems in the kidney or the heart itself.)

THREE FORMS OF CHINESE THERAPY

As we said earlier, Chinese medicine often combines three forms of treatment:

1. Acupuncture and massage

2. Herbal medicine

3. Qi-gong, or energy-releasing exercise.

* Acupuncture and Massage:

The body contains more than one thousand "acupoints" according to Chinese medicine. Each of these areas can be stimulated to enhance the flow of qi. Special needles are inserted into these points to help correct the energy flow of energy. The insertion of the very thin needle is usually painless, except for a mild pinprick. Practitioners are careful to avoid blood vessels and major organs.

Needles may be inserted to a depth of about one-fourth to two inches, depending on a variety of factors, and are left in place for an average time of about 20 minutes. Special herbs called moxa (derived from the herb mugwort are often heated either above or on a specific acupoint.

* Herbs

Herbs are used to reorganize the body constituents (qi, blood, and body fluids) within the meridians and internal organs. Multiple herbs in combinations are used for specific effects. In addition, herbs can be added according to specific symptoms. For instance, diuretic herbs may be prescribed to someone whose high blood pressure is related to water retention.

Herbs are dispensed in many different forms, including pills, tinctures, powders and capsules. Fresh herbs may also be given.

* Qi-Gong

This traditional form of Chinese therapy literally translates as "energy exercises." They work to calm the mind, cultivate inner strength and help maintain the body's natural state of internal balance and harmony.

Some qi-gong exercises are like calisthenic or isometrics, others are meditative stances, while others involve the stimulation of acupressure points. Breathing exercises are also used to bring the body into a state of harmony.

The basic qi-gong posture involves standing with feet apart, knees slightly bent, back straight and arms held in front of the body. You are to imagine holding a "globe of qi" in front of you. This posture is maintained from a few minutes to a half-hour. The desired effect is to improve circulation, warm hands and spread relaxation.

A particular qi-gong for heart problems involves using your right palm to massage over the left part of your chest, in a circle covering the left breast, while silently repeating the sound "Ho." A qualified acupuncturist may also employ this form of massage, using his or her own qi to release yours.

There are also massage points to help angina and heart attacks, for heart failure, for high blood pressure and for arrhythmias. These techniques can be learned for self-care, but it is recommended that they be learned from a qualified acupuncturist.

Licensing requirements differ by state. Some license only M.D.'s aa acupuncturists; other states require separate licenses. Licensed practitioners should have taken a national certification or equivalent exam, while physicians should have completed a minimum of 225 hours of training (according to by the U.N.'s World Health Organization).

AROMATHERAPY: UPDATING AN ANCIENT PRACTICE

Does the odor of a particular food trigger a feeling of comfort? Does the scent of certain flower invoke childhood memories? If so, you're definitely a member of the human species.

The connection between scent, emotion, and memory is universal, and has led to a revival of an ancient form of medical practice known as aromatherapy.

Aromatherapy is a form of natural medicine that uses essential oils derived from the roots, sterns, seeds and flowers to help restore the body's emotional and physical balance. First developed by the ancient Egyptians, aromatherapy is an offshoot of herbal medicine--and now one of the fastest-growing branches of alternative medicine in the United States.

The actual term aromatherapy was devised in the mid-thirties by a French chemist, Rene-Maurice Gattefosse. Gattefosse badly burned his hand during an experiment in his family's perfume factory. Knowing that lavender was used in medicine for burns, he plunged his hand into a vat of pure lavender oil. After his hand healed very quickly, Gattefosse began to explore the healing powers of other essential oils.

Essential oils, which are composed of the plant's most volatile constituents, are extracted through a process of steam distillation or cold pressing. Each essential oil is made up of several different organic molecules that, working together, give the oil its unique perfume as well as its particular therapeutic qualities.

Some essential oils, known to have antiviral and antibacterial properties, can be used to treat infections such as herpes simplex, skin and bowel infections, and the flu. Other types of oils stimulate the body's anti-inflammatory response, making them helpful in treating arthritis and similar conditions.

ESSENTIAL OILS AND THE CARDIOVAS-CULAR SYSTEM

One of the primary risk factors in developing heart disease is excess stress. Stress overstimulates the sympathetic nervous system and the hormonal system, thereby raising blood pressure and heart rate and increasing blood lipid levels.

Inhaling certain essential oils, however, can help to bring the sympathetic nervous system into balance with the actions of the parasympathetic nervous system and thus To understand how, you have to examine first how the brain and body recognize and react to scents. There is a pathway that brings scents from the air directly to your emotions.

This path begins in the nose, where specialized nerve cells first recognize a scent, then pass the information on to other nerve cells. Finally, the sensory information is brought to a part of the central nervous system known as the limbic system.

The limbic system appears also to be the seat of emotions. It stores emotional information and memories that can be triggered by scent--and set off physical reactions, including a rise in blood pressure, heart rate and serum cholesterol levels. Choosing essential oils known to help relax the nervous system, may help reduce the ill effects of stress on the cardiovascular system.

Several essential oils are considered beneficial to the heart and circulatory system. But check with your alternative practitioner before undertaking an extended aromatherapy regimen; essential oils are concentrations of powerful herbs and should be used with care.

* Angelica oil. Angelica oil is derived from a biennial plant whose roots and seeds are stem-distilled to produce a woody-scented oil. Though often used to help soothe indigestion and heal scars and bruises, angelica oil is known to stimulate circulation and remove toxins from the body.

* Anise seed oil. This, also known as sweet cumin, is a tender annual related to parsley and fennel. Aniseed grows in both wild and cultivated states around the Mediterranean, and since colonial times has grown in the United States. Although the main property of anise is digestive, aniseed is also effective in calming heart palpitations.

* Basil oil. Basil is an herb now cultivated around the world. A popular cooking spice, basil is used in aromatherapy to fortify the nervous system and to remedy anxiety or stress, especially when combined with soy oil and rubbed into the body.

* Chamomile oil. For centuries, chamomile and the oil derived from its flowers and roots have been used for medicinal purposes. Until World War II, chamomile oil was used as a natural disinfectant and

antiseptic in hospitals.

It is known to help cure respiratory infections and allergies, as well as soothe indigestion, headaches and menstrual cramps. Because of its relaxing effects, it is also helpful in reducing heart rate and blood pressure.

* Clary sage/sage oil. Made from the flowering tops and leaves of a common perennial plant, chary sage oil has long been used for its medicinal properties. It is an all-around tonic that can help reduce fatigue, irritability, and depression and thus help to bolster self-esteem and reduce overall stress on the body.

* Lavender oil. Used topically, lavender can help heal burns, wounds and insect bites. To benefit patients with stress-related cardiovascular disease, it can help calm the sympathetic nervous system and stimulate the parasympathetic nervous system.

* Marjoram oil. Most often prescribed to reduce stress and anxiety, marjoram oil also increases circulation by dilating the arteries, making it a perfect choice for many people with high blood pressure.

WHERE TO GET ESSENTIAL OILS

An enormous quantity of plant material is needed to make even a small amount of essential. To make an ounce of lavender oil, for instance, requires about 12 pounds of fresh lavender flowers. Fortunately, only a very small amount of oil is needed to have therapeutic effects.

Although it's possible to make essential oils with a homemade still, most people choose to purchase prepared oils from health-food stores and/or mail-order companies.

Warning: The fragrance industries often use toxic and irritating chemicals like hexane, methylene, and benzene to distill essences from flowers and plants. These may be relatively harmless when used in perfume, but essential oils extracted in this way have lost much of their heating qualities. When buying oils to use as aromatherapy, make sure they're labeled "Pure Essential Oils" or "PEO." When used as directed the essential ingredients are safe, but they can cause rashes, abdominal pain and otherunpleasant side effects. Always follow directions and/or consult anaromatherapist for information.

You can buy essential oils in their pure form or already diluted with another base oil, usually made from olives, soy or almonds. In addition, herbs which "fix" the scents are added, so potency is maintained over time.

Combining essences with base oils does not change chemical composition, but will help to reduce their potential toxicity to the skin or internal tissue.

SMELLING AWAY STRESS

There are two main ways to use essential oils as part of your stress-management program to help prevent or reverse heart disease:

1. Inhalants. Just breathing in the odors and minute particles of plant material may help bring your body back into balance. There are several equally effective methods of inhaling essential oils:

* Diffusers: Mechanical devices disperse microparticles of essential oils into the air.

* Facial saunas: Pour boiling water into a bowl,

then add a few drops of essential oil. Drape a towel over your head and lean over the bowl, enclosing both head and bowl. The essences are absorbed both through the skin and nasal membranes.

* Aroma lamps: Putting a few drops of oil on a light bulb or burning a candle under a cup that has drops of oil in it will volatilize the oil into the air, making your whole environment rich with soothing aroma.

2. Topical applications. When diluted properly with base oils, essential oils may be safely and effectively applied directly to the skin.

* Massage: Oils can be massaged into the face, back, chest, or any part of the body that is feeling pain or stress. Massage is an excellent relaxation method.

* Bath oils: Adding a few drops of an essential oil to bath water both adds to the relaxing atmosphere and allows the oils to seep into the skin.

As is true of all forms of natural medicine, however, aromatherapy is highly individualized: Something that relaxes one person may stimulate another. Experimentation with several oils, alone or in combination, may be recommended.

Cautions: You should discuss with your physician and/or natural medicine practitioner how aromatherapy can fit safely into your personal heart disease treatment plan.

Other cautions:

* Check with your doctor. If you are pregnant, check with both your obstetrician and your alternative practitioner before using any essential oils. Do not take essential oils internally unless you first discuss the matter thoroughly with your practitioner.

* Perform a patch test. Before you use any essential oil on your skin, always perform a patch test. To do so, wash about a 2-inch square on your forearm and dry it carefully. Apply a tiny drop of the essential oil, diluting it with an equal part of a bland oil, like olive oil. Then place a Band-Aid over the area and wait 24 hours. If no irritation occurs, use the oil in the formulas. If you develop a rash or are otherwise made to feel uncomfortable, try another oil. A patch test is especially important if you have allergies or particularly sensitive skin.

* Keep essential oils out of your eyes.

* Store essential oils in dark glass or metal bottles and protect them from light and heat.

BIOFEEDBACK: TUNING INTO HEART-HEALTH

Though still considered an alternative medicine by many, biofeedback is rapidly becoming mainstream. It is certainly one of the more scientific methods of revealing and measuring the mind-body connection.

Its potential for treating cardiovascular disease comes in the underlying premise that high blood pressure--and other functions of the autonomic nervous system--can be reduced if the person simply learns to control the bodily responses involved. In other words, when properly trained, you can learn to lower your blood pressure and slow your heart rate by concentrating on doing so with your conscious mind. You will do so by triggering your parasympathetic nervous system to counteract the actions of your sympathetic nervous system during and after times of stress.

Biofeedback was developed when studies showed animals could control their autonomic functions, like blood pressure, by being given a reward or a punishment. Physicians adapted those findings to design ways for humans to consciously control what were once considered unconscious functions.

There are several biofeedback methods, but all have three things in common:

1. They measure a physiological function (such as blood pressure);

2. They convert this measurement to some kind of simple signal (a blinking light, mercury levels in a thermometer, etc.);

3. They feed back this information to the person learning to control his or her body processes.

One biofeedback method involves a monitoring machine equipped with lights similar to traffic lights. A special blood pressure cuff with a microphone projects the sound of any changes in blood pressure.

As pressure rises, the light on the machine, as well as the sounds emitted by the microphone, allow the patient to monitor the blood pressure level. Ideally the patient learns to control his blood pressure by consciously calming down if the pressure is too high, or by thinking about stressful situations if the pressure is too low.

The goal is to continue to control blood pressure, say, or pain from angina, or other symptoms of heart disease without the need for the monitoring machine. Over time, a patient can learn to recognize both the normally automatic physiological changes present with high blood pressure and the stress that triggers it.

Obviously, to be guided through this process a person needs an experienced practitioner. The place to start is with a mainstream or alternative practitioner. He or she can recommend where you can learn the appropriate techniques.

CARDIO-CHIROPRACTIC

Chiropractic is not usually associated with internal organs, only lower back pain and other musculoskeletal disorders. But this growing health care practice has proven to be an effective complementary for a wide range of ailments, including high blood pressure and heart disease.

Chiropractic therapy centers on restoring proper balance and structure to the spinal column and joints. By doing so, it attempts to restore balance to the nervous system, which radiates from the spinal cord to bodily organs and tissues. When the spinal cord is misaligned, it prevents the nervous system from transmitting messages to the muscles, organs and tissues. Pain and/or disease may result.

By keeping the spine in alignment through regular visits to the chiropractor and through proper exercise, you help your body carry out its functions, including healing. Chiropractic, then, can be seen as both treatment for injury and illness and a method of prevention.

However, the causes of heart disease include genetic, environmental and lifestyle factors outside the capacity of chiropractic therapy to alleviate.

So a chiropractor would most likely refer a patient with high blood pressure, coronary artery disease and/or angina to a physician for evaluation and treatment. A nutritionist, herbalist, or other alternative therapist might be recommended for additional support.

Yet chiropractic has proved a useful complementary treatment for cardiovascular disease in several ways:

1. Proper alignment of the spine allows the autonomic nervous system to function properly. The two branches of the autonomic nervous system, the sympathetic and parasympathetic, must work in coordination with each other and with the hormonal system in order for normal blood pressure and heart function to be maintained. The part of the spine most involved with cardiovascular function is the upper cervical region, located in the neck.

2. Adjustment of the midthoracic region of the spine (in the middle of the back) frees the nerves that stimulate kidney function, helping the body eliminate salt and water through more efficient urine production. This lowers blood volume and, hence, blood pressure. Manipulation of the midthoracic region also has an effect on the biochemical activities of the adrenal gland, leading to increased production of the hormone aldosterone, which is essential to proper salt and water retention and excretion.

3. By releasing areas of spinal tension, chiropractic promotes general relaxation. As stress reduction is an essential part of any successful cardiovascular treatment plan, chiropractic is especially useful to anyone with cardiovascular disease.

Again, though chiropractic is not recommended as a first-line treatment for most sufferers of coronary artery disease and/or high blood pressure, it is worth exploring as part of an overall holistic plan to bring your body back to a natural state of balance.

HERBAL MEDICINE: AN ANCIENT ART COMES WEST

In fact, herbal medicine is the most ancient form of health care. It has been used in all societies throughout history. It is a form of medicine just being rediscovered in America, though herbal preparations are widely recommended by doctors in Germany, France and England.

More amazing: Currently, 25 percent of all U.S. prescription drugs are derived from trees, shrubs, or herbs; while other drugs are synthesized to mimic natural plant compounds.

You might think that with this long history, most plants have been studied for their medical applications. But not so. Of the 250,000 to 500,000 different kinds of plants growing on the earth today, only about 5,000 have been investigated.

There are other parallels between herbs and conventional pharmaceutical drugs. Naturally occurring chemicals in herbs work within the body to alter its chemistry. Unlike purified or isolated drugs, however, plants contain a wide variety of substances and, hence, less of any one particular active chemical. This attribute makes plants far less toxic than most manufactured drugs.

Natural herbs have another benefit. They contain substances that work in combination to restore balance to the body. Example: The plant meadowsweet contains compounds similar to those of aspirin--salicylates--which often irritate the stomach lining. But, unlike commercially prepared aspirin, meadowsweet also contains substances that soothe the gastric lining and reduce stomach acidity, thus providing relief from pain while protecting the stomach from irritation.

Like other kinds of alternative therapy, herbal medicine doesn't try to cure disease per se, but rather to help the body remain in, or return to, a state of balance we call "health." To accomplish this, herbalists explore their patients' lifestyle and dietary habits to develop an individualized treatment plan. And they often carry this exploration far beyond where most mainstream physicians would go.

Herbal remedies are also incorporated in types of traditional approaches to medicine and health, including Chinese medicine and Ayurveda. Each of these, however, may use herbs in a slightly different way, depending upon how the body is viewed and the condition diagnosed.

How different herbs act on the body and how they are used to treat specific illnesses:

* Some herbs act best as anti-inflammatories, soothing the symptoms of inflammation or reducing the inflammatory response of the tissue directly.

* Others are effective antimicrobials, helping the body destroy or resist bacteria and viruses.

* Other herbs are used as stimulants for the digestive system.

How Do You Take Herbs?

Herbs are available in many forms, including:

* Capsules and tablets: These allow herbs to be taken quickly and without requiring that you taste them.

* Whole herbs: Plants or plant parts that are dried and either cut or powdered to be used as teas or as cooking herbs.

* Extracts and tinctures: These are made by grinding the roots, leaves and/or flowers of an herb and immersing them in a solution of alcohol and water for a period of time.

HERBS AND HEART DISEASE

Herbs may be employed as part of a holistic approach to the treatment of heart disease, along with proper nutrition, exercise and stress reduction. Herbs that might help the body restore the cardiovascular system to proper working order include those known to be hypotensive (blood- pressure-reducing), diuretic (fluid-reducing), calmative (anxiety-reducing) and tonic (energy-building).

There are, however, no set prescriptions in herbal medicine or in any form of alternative therapy. As for any dietary program, nutritional supplement plan or exercise routine, herbal treatment of a particular heart condition should only be planned by a trained professional after a complete examination and workup--and mainstream diagnosis.

Another key factor herbalists take into consideration is a patient's willingness to accept responsibility for his or her own health.

During a first appointment with an herbalist, you should expect the practitioner to take a complete medical history (including noting what medications and supplements you are taking). Many herbal practitioners also perform a physical exam. One or more natural medications would then be prescribed, designed to strengthen your constitution while alleviating your symptoms.

Herbs for Treatment of Heart Disease:

As part of an overall cardiovascular treatment plan, a qualified herbalist will help the patient plan a healthy diet, suggest nutritional supplements and discuss the need to increase your physical activity and reduce stress. Most herbalists also work well with other health-care professionals, from both mainstream medicine and alternative therapies. It is crucial, in such a case, that all those who care for you are apprised of any treatment you receive.

And remember: Herbs are drugs, often powerful ones. So always let your herbalist know what current medications you are taking and if you are pregnant or breastfeeding, so a safe and effective herbal treatment plan can be tailored for you.

Although your particular body chemistry will indicate what herbs will be most effective for you, the following herbs are the ones most used to treat cardiovascular disease:

* Hawthorn. The berries, flowers and leaves of the hawthorn shrub have been used in folk medicine in Europe and China for centuries. Indeed, they are some of the primary heart tonics in natural medicine. More recently, medical researchers have studied hawthorn for its effects on the cardiovascular system.

Hawthorn berries (like other berries) get their color from substances called flavonoids. Flavonoids, besides being potent antioxidants, dilate coronary blood vessels, lower blood lipids and stabilize arterial walls. They also act to inhibit an enzyme, ACE, which helps create high blood pressure. In fact, they function similarly to the drug captopril, commonly given to combat high blood pressure.

Because hawthorn improves heart muscle metabolism, it can be used to treat congestive heart failure and cardiac arrhythmias. It's also mildly diuretic.

How to take it: Dried hawthorn berries or flowers, 3 to 5 grams, can be taken as capsules or teas three times daily. Infusions can be taken, 1/4 to 1/3 teaspoon three times per day. Hawthorn has a low toxicity.

* Garlic. The oils that give garlic its pungency also reduce LDL cholesterol and raise HDL cholesterol. In Germany, garlic extracts are approved over-the-counter drugs for those with elevated blood lipids. And in India a study matching two populations with identical diets except for garlic showed lower blood lipids in the high-garlic group. Garlic has also been shown to aid in thinning the blood and reducing platelet aggregation, thus reducing the risk of blood clots. Finally, garlic has lowered blood pressure by 10 to 20 points in both human and animal studies.

How to take it: In some studies, 3 to 8 cloves of raw garlic were given daily. Capsules are also available; unfortunately the substance responsible for many of garlic's good effects, called allicin, is also responsible for its strong odor, and capsules with the substances removed do not work as well as whole, fresh garlic. There is some evidence that capsules coated so that they break down low in the intestines work better, and with less odor. About 2 to 6 capsules per day is a common dose.

(See Chapter 11 for more about garlic.)

* Ginseng. Wars have been fought in the Orient over ginseng. But this herb is actually several different substances. Korean or Chinese ginseng is the most

famous, known to reduce blood clot formation, reverse oxidation and lower blood lipids. Its effect on blood pressure, however, is peculiar: In low doses it seems to raise blood pressure, while lowering pressure in higher doses. But the main use of ginseng is in helping to cope with stress, by improving adrenal gland function.

Siberian ginseng also improves adrenal function and lowers lipids, and seems to bring both high and low blood pressure closer to normal ranges.

How to take it: Perhaps the most popular way to take either type of ginseng is as a tea or infusion made by stirring about 1/2 teaspoon of powdered ginseng into a cup of hot water (three times a day).

At a Chinese herbal pharmacy you can pay $200 or more for a piece of Chinese ginseng root (price is related to the potency). A reasonably priced root ($10 to $15 range) can be sliced into 2 to 6 gram pieces (about 2 square inches) and cooked as tea.

Warning: Too much high-potency ginseng can be toxic.

* Ginkgo biloba. The leaves of this tree, the oldest species in the world, contain special flavonoids which give the plant both its characteristic smell and its remarkable vascular effects. Ginkgo has been shown to increase arterial blood flow in a variety of situations, including cerebral vascular insufficiency and stroke, hardening of the peripheral arteries, impotence due to lack of blood flow, and in cardiac problems. Ginkgo also keeps blood platelets from sticking and breaking down and increases oxygen supply to the arteries and veins.

More on Ginkgo and Circulatory Disorders:

A 1965 study reported that ginkgo biloba extract lowered blood pressure and dilated or expanded the peripheral blood vessels, including capillaries in 10 patients with post-thrombotic syndrome. This did not increase capillary permeability but it did reduce the swelling.

In 1972 the use of ginkgo biloba extract (GBE) was compared with other vasodilators, notably hydrogenated alkaloids of ergot, acetylcholine chloride and sodium nicotinate. All patients had varying degrees of vascular disease.

The research team stated that the vasodilator action of GBE is similar to the other substances but is significantly more constant.

A study in 1977 was conducted to determine the activity of GBE on cerebral blood flow in 20 patients, ages 62 to 85, who were diagnosed with cerebral circulatory insufficiency, due to age and hardening of the arteries.

The patients were treated orally and intramuscularly for 15 days. Because of the age and health of the volunteers, the researchers maintained low dosages of GBE and did not expect spectacular results. However, they reported that the cerebral blood flow was much improved in 15 of the cases.

In another 1977 study researchers reported functional improvement in 65 percent of patients with arterial leg disease following GBE therapy. There was only a 22.5 percent response in the placebo group. Some patients in the treatment group also reported better circulation to the extremities and a lessening of impotence, among other things.

About two-thirds of the patients receiving GBE showed definite clinical improvement, compared with

16 percent given a placebo, when treated for a variety of peripheral vascular diseases.

GBE enhances blood flow not only through the large blood vessels, but also small vessels like the capillaries close to the skin. A 1992 test at the

University of Saarland in Hamburg, Germany, revealed that GBE increases microcirculation through the capillaries of the body. The study involved 10 patients whose skin microcirculation was monitored every 30 minutes. The results showed a 57 percent increase in blood flow through the capillaries of the finger after one hour.

Safety

All clinical indications so far are for very low toxicity or side effects from using ginkgo biloba extract, except for minor reversible gastric disturbances.

A more recent study in 1989 conducted at several research centers and hospitals involving 8,505 persons observed over six months reported that the total occurrence of adverse effects was 0.4 percent. All of these were minor and temporary. Once again, gastric disturbances were the most common, totaling 0.1 percent. Thus, ginkgo extracts have proven to be quite safe.

How to take it: A standard amount of ginkgo biloba extract (GBE) is usually 40 mg. taken three times a day. Higher dosages are not recommended.

* Guggul. The Indian mukul myrrh tree has a resin shown to lower cholesterol and triglycerides as well as or better than the common drugs on the market, and without toxicity. It works by increasing the liver's metabolism of LDL cholesterol.

How to take it: The common form of gugulipid is

an extract with 4 percent guggulsterone (the active component). A common dosage is 500 mg. three times per day.

* Coleus. This decorative plant has for centuries been studied for its cardiovascular effects. It relaxes smooth muscles, which makes it useful for treating high blood pressure and angina. It also increases the force of heart contractions, doubling its positive effect.

How to take it: Same as for hawthorn. In fact, the two herbs are often used in combination to treat cardiovascular conditions. Coleus has very low toxicity.

* Ginger. Ginger has not only been shown to lower cholesterol, but has a tonic effect on the heart.

How to take it: Ginger can be cooked in foods, taken in tea or in capsule form 2 to 3 times a day.

* European mistletoe. In Europe there are many blood-pressure-lowering herbal preparations containing mistletoe on the market.

How to take it: Since European mistletoe can be toxic, it's usually administered in small amounts (1/2 to 1 teaspoon of the dried herb) combined with hawthorn and other herbs.

* Cayenne. This spice, which is also sold under the name capsicum, has been called food for the heart. In fact, cayenne is one of the most effective general tonics for the body. It stimulates blood flow and strengthens the heartbeat.

How to take it: Capsicum capsules are available in most health-food stores. But if you want to make an infusion, pour a cup of boiling water onto 1/2 to 1 teaspoon of the herb and let it stand for 10 minutes. A tablespoon of this should be mixed with hot water and drunk.

* Bilberry. This berry contains the same flavonoids as hawthorn and many of the same beneficial effects. Bilberry seems to particularly helpful in strengthening circulation. For this reason, it is often recommended for treatment of varicose veins and thrombophlebitis.

How to take it: Bilberry, being nontoxic, can be used liberally, dried in tea or fluid extracts in the doses given for hawthorn.

* Khella. An article in the New England Journal of Medicine in 1951 supported the use of this plan in angina pectoralis. Specifically, Khella appears to be helpful in increasing the amount of exercise a person can tolerate before experiencing angina.

How to take it: Standard doses would be 250 to 300 mg. of the extract (containing 12 percent of the active component khellin). Higher doses can cause side effects.

* Angelica. Various types of angelica are used to treat angina, high blood pressure, poor circulation and arrhythmias. Angelica can be grown in a home garden, if the soil is moist and the area partly shaded.

How to take it: Angelica, which has low toxicity, is usually prescribed in the same dose as khella.

* Chamomile. This is probably the best known and most widely used herbal medicine. It has been shown to promote relaxation and reduce stress in people with heart disease.

How to take it: Chamomile tea is made by pouring a cup of boiling water over two or three teaspoonsful of dried leaves and letting it stand for five to ten minutes.

* Grape seed extract. This extract, which the

active ingredient "proanthocyanidin," has been shown to have antioxidant effects. Of particular benefit to those with cardiac conditions, grape seed extract may reduce oxidation of lipoproteins--one of the first steps in the formation of cholesterol plaque.

   * Foxglove (Digitalis). This is plant from which the widely used cardiac medication, digitalis, comes. But foxglove is considered too dangerous for home use. In fact, unless your medical herbalist is specifically trained to use this substance, foxglove should be avoided.

HOMEOPATHY AND CARDIOVASCULAR DISEASE

   Heart disease and high blood pressure are usually chronic conditions. In most cases they result from long-term deficiencies, lifestyle-poor diets, lack of exercise, or high stress levels.

   Because of this, they are candidates for treatment by what are called "holistic" therapies. These involve working to restore proper balance to an individual's own internal environment.

   Homeopathy is a branch of holistic medicine. Perhaps you are interested in exploring it. If so, do not stop taking any cardiovascular medication until you first check with your mainstream physician.

   Origins of Homeopathy

   The term "homeopathy" is derived from the Greek "homoios" (meaning "similar") and "pathos" ("suffering"). Is it a fringe practice? Far from it.

   The World Health Organization estimates that

some 500 million people around the world now use homeopathy as a treatment for disease.

Its proponents and practitioners believe that a physician's role should be to help a patient's own body heal itself and that true heating cannot take place by simply administering chemicals to override the body's natural processes.

They believe in a "vital force," a life power that animates and rules the body, keeping it in balance and health. Disease occurs, according to holistic medicine, when a disturbance of this vital force takes place.

To a homeopath, a "disease" then consists of symptoms produced by the body in its own efforts to heal itself. To help the body in that process--to strengthen the vital force against the illness-a homeopath administers remedies designed to match these symptoms, not to alleviate them as Western medicine is designed to do.

This principle is known as the Law of Similars, or "like cures like." By making symptoms temporarily worse, a remedy attempts to strengthen the body's own power to heal itself. In the view of homeopathy, any therapy that tries to suppress symptoms actually prolongs the underlying disturbance.

Another homeopathic theory is the Law of Infinitesimals. This theory states that the smaller the dose of medicine, the greater its potency and effect on the body's vita) force. Homeopathic remedies are extracts derived by soaking plant, animal, mineral, or other biological material in alcohol to form what is known as the mother tincture. This tincture is again diluted with alcohol, shaken vigorously, then diluted again.

This process of shaking and diluting, repeated

several times, is known as succussion. Many researchers believe that through succussion the vital energy of a substance is transferred to the tincture-- even though there appears to be no trace of the original herb or mineral left. The resulting solution is added to tablets, usually made of sugar, then ingested by the patient.

Homeopathic medicines, however, are only prescribed after a careful evaluation of a patient's particular set of symptoms and physical and emotional make-up.

How a homeopath treats a disease depends entirely on an individual's particular pattern of symptoms. While a conventional physician will offer everyone with angina pains the same treatment (usually beta blockers or calcium-channel blockers), a homeopath recognizes several different symptom patterns associated with angina and has remedies for each one.

It's not possible to describe how a homeopath would diagnose or treat someone with cardiovascular disease, since therapy is based on individual needs and symptoms. In fact, a homeopath may consider the source of cardiovascular disease not to be the heart or the vessels, but an imbalance elsewhere in the body or mind. Like many other forms of holistic medicine homeopathy sees the emotional and intellectual health of an individual as a critical factor in physical health.

Generally speaking, however, homeopathic remedies for cardiovascular disease might include the following:

* Aconitum napellus; Also known as wolfsbane or monkshood, this perennial herb contains aconitine, a deadly poison. When succussed to a homeopathic

dose, however, aconiturn appears to slow pulse and calm breathing, making it a suitable treatment for individuals whose cardiovascular disease may be due to excess stress.

* Arnica montana: This herb grows in the mountains of Europe and the northwestern United States. It is known to reduce high blood pressure and to help resolve other heart disorders.

* Belladonna: Also called deadly nightshade, belladonna contains atropine, a potent central nervous system stimulant. Under careful supervision, belladonna may be prescribed to a patient with high blood pressure.

* Calcarea carbonica: Calcarea is made from oyster shells and has a high calcium content. It is often indicated when the calcium metabolism is imbalanced, thus affecting the blood pressure.

The homeopathic treatment for any disorder, including cardiovascular disease, requires continuing observation and, in some cases, a series of different remedies prescribed on the basis of new, emerging symptoms.

Warning: We strongly recommend that anyone interested in homeopathy thoroughly research the subject before pursuing it in preference to treatment from a mainstream physician.

HEARTY MEDITATION TECHNIQUES

Meditation is used in many religious disciplines as a method of spiritual awakening. But it's also effective both in reducing general stress and in directly improving cardiovascular health. As with other relaxation methods, meditation quiets the sympathetic nervous system, thereby reducing the heart rate, breathing, blood pressure and muscle tension. And these beneficial effects may last for hours after the meditation session.

Meditation can also help you focus on the cause of your stress and to change the way you respond to the challenges you face. By mastering meditative techniques, an individual can improve the sense of control over not only blood pressure but other aspects of physical and psychosocial life. Many who meditate find they are able to sleep more deeply, stop smoking more easily and recover more quickly from stress.

Basic Meditation Technique

Here is a simple meditation exercise that can help promote relaxation.

Find a quiet place. Wear comfortable, loose clothing. Sit on the floor in a comfortable position, or in a straight-backed chair. Rest your hands on your legs.

Lower your eyelids so your eyes are almost closed. Take a deep breath, exhale slowly. Count your breaths.

Inhale. count one. Exhale, count two. Inhale, count three. Exhale, count four. Do this to ten, and then start again with one. Try this for 5 minutes every day for a week. Gradually increase the time to 30 minutes a day.

Meditation for relaxation requires no special training, and can be done at any time of day, in any comfortable space. All it takes is several minutes to an hour of uninterrupted quiet.

CARDIOVASCULAR EFFECTS OF YOGA

Yoga used to be an exotic enigma to most Westerners, associated with strange, mystical practices. Most of picture a yoga practitioner sitting in a "full lotus" position, lighting incense and chanting "Om." And while there exist mystical and philosophical schools of yoga, there are also many kinds which emphasize physical culture.

In fact, some believe yoga to be the most complete form of exercise in the world.

Yoga exercises are a part of Hatha Yoga, the Yoga of the Physical (in Sanskrit, "Hatha Yoga" means "Sun-Moon Union"). These movements emphasize the slow stretching of muscles, and are especially useful in promoting flexibility and increased circulation.

There is an obvious similarity between many of the Yoga exercises (or asanas) and plain old calisthenics. The main difference is in the way they are done. Instead of the old rapid movements typical of calisthenics, Yoga postures and movements are slow and measured (similar to those in Chinese tai-chi). One basic reason is to teach muscular control and mental concentration.

For more information: There is no shortage of good introductions to Yoga exercises. Check your local library or bookstore. Better yet, your local YMCA or YWCA probably offers a course in Yoga for health.

And there's another source. The ancient discipline has been enjoying new popularity these days, and, in response, a spate of new yoga videos has hit the market.

Tapes are available for all levels, from beginners to old hands. Phone numbers are given for independent releases that might be hard to find. Other videos can be ordered from local video stores.

* "Yoga with Linda Arkin for Flexibility"; "Yoga with Linda Arkin for Relaxation and Rejuvenation"; "Yoga with Linda Arkin for Strength," WarnerVision, $9.95.

There is little here a beginner can't tackle. Each tape is 45 minutes.

* "New Yoga Basics," and "New Yoga Challenge," WarnerVision, $19.95 each.

These accompnay Kathy Smith's best-selling "New Yoga" video. "Basics" is for beginners. "Challenge" is for those with more strength and flexibility.

* "Yoga Alignment and Form" with John Friend, Delphi Productions, $29.95 plus $4.40 shipping and handling, (800) 331-6839. In 90 minutes, Houston-based John Friend explains the intricacies of iyengar yoga, which emphasizes form and alignment. Not for beginners. The video comes with a 45-page booklet detailing concepts and poses.

* "Yoga with Richard Freeman," Delphi Productions, $29.95 plus $4.50 shipping and handling, (800) 331-6939. A serious program of ashtanga yoga, popular among pop-yoga practitioners these days--it's also being called power yoga for its fast movement and aerobic qualities. Two hours plus a 96-page booklet.

* "The Sivananda Yoga Video Learning Package," ABA Video, $24.95, (212) 874-2217. Filmed in the Sivananda Yoga Retreat in the Bahamas, the

lesson is in six parts: an explanation of yoga principals; a demonstration of a sequence of hatha yoga poses along with descriptions of their benefits; brief instructions for doing each pose; breathing exercises; a follow-along class; meditation techniques; and relaxation. Includes an audio-tape class for beginners and an instructional booklet.

* "Bryan Kest's Power Yoga Series," Warner Home Video, $14.95 each.

Three-tape series, low key and encouraging approach to three challenging ashtanga yoga workouts. It helps to know a little about rudimentary yoga poses before trying these.

AYURVEDA: YOGIC MEDICINE

Often linked to yoga is an ancient Indian philosophy of health known as Ayurveda. It is no antique, however, but a vital teaching followed by millions of people around the world. The Sanskrit word Ayurveda means "the science of life and longevity."

Like Chinese medicine and holistic medicine, Ayurvedic teaching sees each individual person as an extension of the universe, and health as a state of balance within the body and between the body and the universe. In Ayurveda, there is no dividing line between body, mind, and spirit, and disease can be caused by physical, psychological, or spiritual imbalances. If one's mind and spirit are in harmony, so will the body be healthy. But if conflict is prevalent, the physical self will descend into disease. Since disease involves both physical and spiritual factors, so does treatment require both levels.

Ayurveda also views disease as an opportunity to

reexamine our spiritual and physical lives in order to correct imbalances. Disease, therefore, is a "healthy" way to bring us closer to what is known as the cosmic consciousness.

The life force, known as "qi" in Chinese medicine, is called "prana" in Ayurveda. Prana is the animating power of life. Ayurveda also teaches that within each of us is a divine healer, a cosmic consciousness, that, i properly directed, can restore our balance and energy. Treatment of disease in

Ayurvedic medicine seeks to strengthen and direct that individual cosmicconsciousness.

Balance and harmony, according to Ayurvedic principles, are governed by three "doshas"--energy forces that act on the substances and organs within the body. When the doshas are balanced, the body can function harmoniously, resulting in good health. When the doshas become imbalanced, disease results.

Ayurvedic tradition also believes that each individual also has a specific body type--also called a dosha. Your dosha is determined by body shape, personality and other qualities. Once an Ayurvedic practitioner determines your dosha, he or she can prescribe the right kind of diet, exercise and routines to keep you in optimal health. An unbalanced dosha or doshas create emotional or mental disorders as well as physical problems.

In fact, the main cause of disease, according to Ayurvedic medicine, is said to be "failure of intelligence," or prajnaparadha. This lack of understanding of the natural harmony of life can result from fear, desire, greed or other destructive forces.

Types of dosha:

1. "Vata" activates the physical system and is responsible for breathing and the circulation of blood. The seats of vata are the large intestine, pelvic cavity, skin, ears and thighs. Organs associated with vata include bones, brain (especially motor activity), heart and lungs.

Those who are predominantly a vata type tend to be thin, with prominent features and cool, dry skin. They may have a rapid speech pattern and a feeble pulse. Vatas tend to be moody and vivacious and have active, creative minds.

They are prone to anxiety and disorders of the vata organs. Vata's season is autumn--a dry, windy season during which vata people tend to develop arthritis, rheumatism and constipation.

2. The "kapha" dosha holds together the structure of body and is located in the chest, lungs and spinal fluid. Organs include brain (primarily information storage), joints, lymph and stomach. Those with a predominant kapha body type tend to be heavyset and have cool, oily skin. Kaphas are often very relaxed and tolerant people, slow to anger but with a tendency to procrastinate.

Kapha types are prone to obesity, and thus to heart disease, as well as to illnesses of the kapha organs, such as allergies and sinus problems. The kapha season is winter, when the respiratory system is particularly susceptible to colds and congestion.

3. "Pitta" governs the metabolic processes of cells. Organs associated include blood, brain (especially memory and learning), hormones (when stimulating activity), liver, small intestine and spleen. Pitta body types tend to have a medium build, thin hair and warm, ruddy skin. Pittas are organized, work hard and

have regular sleeping and eating habits. Although generally warm and loving, a pitta may also display quick bursts of temper.

Pittas tend to suffer from acne, hemorrhoids and ulcers, and may often feel warm and thirsty. Pitta season is summer, and disorders include rashes, diarrhea and other inflammatory conditions.

AYURVEDIC MEDICINE AND HEART DISEASE

In Ayurvedic as well as Chinese medicine, the heart, not the brain, is the seat of consciousness. Thus heart disease often reflects deep-seated issues of identity, feeling and consciousness that we hold inside of us. Causes of heart disease, according to Ayurvedic tradition, may include a wrong diet, physical or emotional trauma, suppressed emotions or excess anxiety.

Heart disease can occur with any of the three doshas. Vata heart disease is indicated by palpitations and tightness in the chest and feelings of restlessness, fear and anxiety. People who experience pitta heart disease may feel flushed, have nosebleeds and vomit sour fluids. Psychologically, people who have pitta heart disease feel angry and irritable and may suffer bursts of temper that aggravate other symptoms. Kapha types, on the other hand, may experience heart disease as a heaviness in the chest, develop a stubborn cough and are often tired.

Treatment of all types of heart disease is dependent upon the emotional spiritual and physical attributes of each individual. But some general prescriptions include:

1. Relaxation and meditation.

The first step toward health involves a period of physical, spiritual and emotional rest. Many people find that meditation and yoga exercises help bring them in touch with their true heart's desires.

2. Detoxification. The first step in this process are to eliminate cigarette smoking, alcohol and environmental pollutants. Other detoxification methods are undertaken only under supervision.

3. Diet. In addition to prescribing a diet to help restore dosha imbalance, an Ayurvedic practitioner may recommend foods rich in antioxidants, such as vitamins C and E and beta-carotene. They may also recommend adding onions and garlic to your diet. Specific dietary recommendations are based on dosha type.

4. Herbal remedies. As we've noted earlier, there are many herbs to strengthen the heart. Practitioners will recommend different herbs depending upon specific dosha imbalance and suspected cause.

To choose Ayurvedic medicine to treat heart disease would most likely necessitate significant changes in eating and exercise habits--and in spiritual outlook. Those who are interested should really study Ayurvedic philosophy.

MEDITATING YOUR WAY TO LOW BLOOD PRESSURE

Those who suffer from hypertension, or high blood pressure, are often counseled to relax. The next question is:

How.

One new way, based on an ancient Hindu practice, may be to meditate. Although hypertension may not always be caused by stress, practicing a form of meditation often used as a relaxation technique can be amazingly effective in controlling it.

In this particular study, Transcendental Meditation outperformed two other frequently recommended nonmedical methods for reducing unhealthy pressures. Among 111 African-American men and women 55 to 85, T.M. was shown to be significantly better at lowering blood pressure than progressive muscle relaxation and instruction on healthier living habits. The findings were reported in the August, 1996, journal Hypertension, published by the American Heart Association.

The blood pressure reductions found in the patients randomly assigned to practice T.M. daily were similar to those commonly achieved with antihypertensive drugs. In long-term drug studies, such reductions have been associated with about 35 percent fewer strokes and heart attacks. The researchers said the findings were particularly impressive because all participants had multiple risk factors for hypertension, including obesity, high alcohol intake, high-sodium diets, low levels of exercise and high levels of psychological stress. The findings indicated that relaxation induced by T.M. can decrease blood pressure even in people who are not under unusual stress, as well as In those with other major hypertension risk factors.

T.M. was not compared in the study to other forms of meditation. For instance, another popular technique--practicing the relaxation response--was devised by Dr. Herbert Benson, a cardiologist affiliated with Harvard

University Medical School. Dr. Benson describes

his technique as a "demystified form of meditation" in which practitioners choose a soothing word and sit quietly focusing upon it twice a day for 10 minutes at a time. The relaxation response has also been shown to lower blood pressure significantly.

Dr. William Sheppard, the study's project director, said he expected that other forms of meditation, like Zen or yoga, would have beneficial effects on blood pressure as well, but that until they were studied scientifically, it was not possible to say which method was most effective.

T-M., which grew out of an ancient Indian practice, allows a person to achieve deep physiological relaxation while remaining awake and alert. It involves sitting quietly with eyes closed for about 20 minutes at a time while the mind focuses on a single soothing sound, or mantra. The technique was brought to the West about 40 years ago by the Maharishi Mahesh Yogi, founder of the Maharishi University of Management in Fairfield, Iowa.

Dr. Charles N. Alexander, a Harvard-trained psychologist and a professor at the Maharishi University who is the lead author of the new study, said that

T.M. Involved only a one-time cost and could have lifelong benefits without causing any unwanted side effects. The technique is taught at T.M. centers in major cities throughout the country at a cost of $600 for students and $1,000 for adults, he said.

Dr. Alexander predicted that the regular practice of T.M. should allow many people with hypertension to avoid lifelong treatments with costly pressure-reducing medications, which can cause side effects like dizziness, impotence and higher cholesterol levels,

However, Dr. Edward D. Frohlich, the journal's

editor, cautioned that patients who choose to practice T.M. and whose blood pressure is currently controlled by medication should continue taking the prescribed drug unless told to stop by their physicians. He added that the study's results might not apply to all patients.

The new study was run under Dr. Sheppard's direction at the Hypertension and Stress Management Research Clinic of West Oakland Health Center in California. Dr. Sheppard, who regularly practices T.M. and similar techniques, said in an interview that while there was still wariness about these mind-body, approaches in the medical community, "attitudes are changing because," many physicians realize that what they have to offer isn't so hot."

Accordingly, the National Institutes of Health has allocated $3 million for two further studies of the long-term effects of T.M., comparing It with other behavioral techniques for the ability to reduce blood pressure, stress and heart disease in African-Americans, who are twice as likely as Caucasian

Americans to develop high blood pressure.

In the study just published, Dr. Alexander said, "T.M. was twice as effective" over all in lowering blood pressure as progressive muscle relaxation, which in turn was much more effective than instruction on healthier habits. While as many as half the patients on prescribed anti-hypertensives fail to take them regularly, Dr. Alexander said, 80 percent of the study's T.M. participants who were followed up five years later were still practicing it.

In the study, conducted over an initial period of three months, women in the T.M. group had an average reduction in systolic blood pressure that was 10.4 points deeper, and a drop in diastolic blood pressure that was 5.9 points deeper, than women getting instruction in improved living habits. For men, the comparable differences were 12.7 points in systolic pressure and 8.1 points in diastolic pressure. Progressive muscle relaxation reduced only diastolic pressure in the men and did not produce statistically significant reductions in blood pressure in the women.

CHORTLE YOUR WAY TO HEART HEALTH

Yogic breathing, progressive relaxation, biofeedback and meditation are useful alternative techniques for reducing stress. But there is one more, very common, very popular, very helpful.

And it's a technique that you should have no trouble finding time to do--laughing. (We discussed this earlier in chapter 6, "10 Easy Things to Reduce Stress.")

Yes, laughter really is one of the best medicines known to humanity. On aphysical level, it increases muscular activity, respiratory activity, oxygen exchange, heart rate and the production of endorphins. Then comes a relaxedstate in which respiration, heart rate, blood pressure and muscle tensionrebound to below normal levels.

Humor's psychological effects are equally beneficial. It provides ahealthy outlet for hostility, an escape from often unpleasant reality and relief from anxiety and tension. If you can laugh at the world, and yourself,you'll find your heart is lighter and your stress less.

DARE TO TAKE CHARGE OF YOUR HEART HEALTH

Remember, whatever types of mainstream or natural therapies you may choose to treat cardiovascular disease, the fundamental ingredients of any successful treatment plan are diet, exercise, and relaxation.

And the person who will make the ultimate difference in any treatment is not the practitioner or therapist but you.

For nobody can really make the optimum changes for you--but you. Nobody can desire it enough, but you.

But do you dare to take your own life in your hands?

You're already doing it, if you think about it. It's all you can do. So do the best you know how, and above all, since it's playing with life, be sure to have a lot of fun along the way.

CALORIE, FAT, CHOLESTEROL, AND SODIUM
CONTENT OF COMMONLY USED FOODS

Food	Amount	Kcal	Fat (gm)	Chol (mg)	Sodium (mg)
Apple, fresh	1 medium	80	0	0	1
juice	1/2 cup	60	0	0	1
Applesauce, canned,					
sweetened	1/2 cup	105	0	0	3
unsweetened	1/2 cup	50	0	0	2
Apricots, fresh	3 small	50	0	0	1
canned, sweet	1/2 cup (4 halves)	100	0	0	1
dried	1/4 cup (4 halves)	80	0	0	9
nectar	1/2 cup	70	0	0	0
Asparagus, fresh	1/2 cup	20	0	0	1
canned, sweet	1/2 cup	20	0	0	235
Avacado, fresh	1/2 med.	190	18	0	15
dip (guacamole)	1/2 cup	140	13	0	165
Banana, fresh	1 6-inch	100	0	0	1
Bacon, cooked	2 slices	109	10	16	303
bits	1 tbsp.	36	2	0	432
Canadian	1 slice	65	4	10	442
Baking powder	1 tsp.	4	0	0	405
Baking soda	1 tsp.	0	0	0	821
Bean dip	1 tbsp.	20	1	2	177
Bean sprouts	1 cup	35	0	0	5
Beans	1/2 cup	118	0	0	7

New And Natural Ways To Your Lower Blood Pressure, Cholesterol And Stress

Food	Amount	Kcal	Fat (gm)	Chol (mg)	Sodium (mg)
baked	1/2 cup	190	6	0	485
garbanzo, cooked	1/2 cup	134	2	0	6
green, cooked	1/2 cup	15	0	0	2
kidney, canned	1/2 cup	112	0	0	4
navy, cooked	1/2 cup	88	0	0	0
pinto, cooked	1/2 cup	92	0	0	0
pork and beans, cooked	1/2 cup	160	4	1	59
refried beans	1/2 cup	230	12	0	340
Beef					
barbecued sandwich with bun	1	509	37	81	506
brisket, baked	3 ounces	367	33	80	46
barbecued	3 ounces	382	34	80	176
Chicken fried steak	4 ounces	370	22	130	350
chop suey	1 cup	300	17	64	1052
chuck roast, baked	3 ounces	240	17	60	40
corned beef	3 ounces	372	30	83	1740
flank steak	3 ounces	158	5	50	47
hamburger patty, broiled	3 ounces	190	10	50	60
jerky	1 piece	38	2	10	418
liver, fried	3 ounces	200	9	255	155
meatloaf	3 ounces	171	11	50	555
pate	1 tbsp.	41	14	40	91
pot pie	1 piece	443	24	41	1008
prime rib, baked	3 ounces	380	33	80	40
round steak	3 ounces	220	13	60	60
short ribs	1 rib	290	24	24	39
sirloin steak, broiled	3 ounces	330	27	80	50
stew	1 cup	220	11	63	90
stroganoff	1 cup	470	33	130	860
sweetbreads	3 ounces	143	3	466	0
tenderloin (fillet)	3 ounces	1741	8	72	54
Beet greens, cooked	1/2 cup	5	0	0	55
Beets, canned	1/2 cup	30	0	0	200
Beverages					
beer	12 ounces	150	0	0	25
beer, non-alcoholic	12 ounces	65	0	0	0

New And Natural Ways To Your Lower Blood Pressure, Cholesterol And Stress

Food	Amount	Fat Kcal	Chol (gm)	Sodium (mg)	(mg)
club soda	6 ounces	0	0	0	30
coffee	1 cup	3	0	0	2
Gatorade	1 cup	39	0	0	123
ginger ale	12 ounces	105	0	0	4
Kool Aid	1 cup	100	0	0	1
lemonade	1 cup	110	0	0	1
mineral water	1 cup	0	0	0	5
quinine water	1 cup	74	0	0	16
soft drinks, all					
canned	12 ounces	150	0	0	10-30
Tang	1 cup	135	0	0	17
tea	1 cup	3	0	0	0
tonic water	12 ounces	132	0	0	0
V-8 juice	6 ounces	31	0	0	364
whiskey	1 1/2 oz.	107	0	0	0
wine	4 ounces	85	0	0	5
Blackberries, fresh	1 cup	80	0	0	2
Blackeyed peas,					
canned	3/4 cup	81	0	0	2
dried, cooked	1 cup	72	1	0	2
Blueberries, fresh	1 cup	90	0	0	960
Bouillon cube	1 cube	18	1	0	10
low-sodium	1 cube	18	1	0	260
Bread					
bagel	1 piece	180	2	0	270
biscuit	1 piece	90	3	2	115
diet	1 slice	40	0	0	100
breadstick	1 piece	23	0	0	265
cornbread	1 piece	180	6	3	190
cornbread muffin	1 2-inch	130	4	2	270
croissant	1 piece	180	11	48	1360
croutons	2 cups	359	1	0	203
English muffin	1 muffin	138	1	0	145
French bread	1 slice	70	0	0	103
mixed grain bread	1 slice	64	1	0	53
pita pocket	1 pita	170	2	0	110
popover	1 medium	112	5	74	90
raisin bread	1 slice	65	0	1	140

New And Natural Ways To Your Lower Blood Pressure, Cholesterol And Stress

Food	Amount	Kcal	Fat (gm)	Chol (mg)	Sodium (mg)
roll, dinner	1 small	85	2	1	140
hard	1 small	160	2	0	315
whole wheat	1 small	90	1	0	197
rye bread	1 slice	65	0	1	140
sweet roll	1 medium	270	16	46	240
white bread	1 slice	70	0	1	130
whole wheat bread	1 slice	65	0	1	130
Brocolli, cooked	1/2 cup	20	0	0	8
raw	1 cup	24	0	0	24
Brussel sprouts	1/2 cup	30	0	0	8
Butter, regular	1 tsp.	35	4	13	40
unsalted	1 tsp.	36	4	11	0
Cabbage, cooked	1/2 cup	15	0	0	10
Cake, (1 piece)					
angel food	1/12 cake	135	0	0	60
brownie without icing	2- inch x 2- inch	146	10	25	75
cheesecake, plain	1/12 cake	255	13	60	170
chocolate cake with icing	1/12 cake	379	16	62	322
cupcake with icing	1	190	6	54	160
fruitcake	1/30 cake	55	2	0	21
gingerbread	2- inch x 2- inch	170	5	0	190
pound cake	1/17 cake	140	9	482	35
Candy, caramels	3 pieces	120	3	2	65
chocolate chips	2 tbsp.	148	8	2	64
fudge	1 ounce	120	5	5	50
gum	1 piece	9	0	0	0
gum drop, small	2 tbsp.	100	0	25	10
hard candy	1 ounce	110	0	0	10
jelly beans	1/4 cup	66	0	0	0
milk chocolate	1.65 ounces	140	9	9	25
peanut brittle	1 ounce	120	3	31	10
peanut butter cup	1 piece	130	8	0	75
Cantaloupe	1/4 melon	50	0	0	20
Carrots, cooked	1/2 cup	20	0	0	25
Cauliflower, cooked	1/2 cup	15	0	0	10

New And Natural Ways To Your Lower Blood Pressure, Cholesterol And Stress

Food	Amount	Fat Kcal	Chol (gm)	Sodium (mg)	(mg)
Celery, raw	1 stalk	15	0	0	100
Cereals					
All Bran	1 cup	210	2	0	960
Alpha Bits	1 cup	119	0	0	227
bran	1 cup	120	2	0	60
Bran Buds	1 cup	210	2	0	516
bran flakes	1 cup	127	0	0	363
Cheerios	1 cup	89	1	0	297
corn flakes	1 cup	95	0	0	325
Cream of Wheat, cooked	1/2 cup	50	0	0	175
granola	1 cup	503	20	0	232
Grape Nuts	1 cup	402	0	0	299
Malt-O-Meal, cooked	1/2 cup	61	0	0	1
oat bran, dry	1/3 cup	110	2	0	0
oatmeal cooked	1/2 cup	69	1	0	218
Product 19	1 cup	126	0	0	386
Puffed Rice	1 cup	54	0	0	1
Puffed Wheat	1 cup	50	0	0	1
Raisin Bran	1 cup	155	1	0	293
Ralston, cooked	1/2 cup	67	0	0	2
Rice Chex	1 cup	110	0	0	240
Rice Krispies	1 cup	112	0	0	340
Shredded Wheat	1 cup	180	1	0	2
Special K	1 cup	76	0	0	154
Sugar Crisp	1 cup	121	0	0	29
Sugar Pops	1 cup	109	0	0	103
Team flakes	1 cup	109	1	0	175
Total	1 cup	109	1	0	352
wheat flakes	1 cup	100	0	0	310
wheat germ	1/3 cup	120	4	0	0
Cheese					
American	1 ounce	110	9	50	405
blue cheese	1 ounce	100	8	21	395
Brie	1 ounce	95	8	28	178
Camembert	1 ounce	85	7	20	239
cheddar	1 ounce	115	10	28	175

New And Natural Ways To Your Lower Blood Pressure, Cholesterol And Stress

Food	Amount	Fat Kcal	Chol (gm)	Sodium (mg)	(mg)
colby	1 ounce	112	9	27	171
cottage cheese,					
regular	1/2 cup	120	5	24	455
low-fat	1/2 cup	81	1	12	459
cream cheese	2 tbsp.	100	10	32	85
Edam	1 ounce	101	7	25	274
feta	1 ounce	75	6	25	316
Gouda	1 ounce	101	8	32	232
gruyere	1 ounce	117	9	31	95
low-calorie cheese	1 ounce	52	2	5	606
low-cholesterol cheese	1 ounce	110	9	5	150
Monterey jack	1 ounce	106	9	26	152
mozzarella, part-skim	1 ounce	72	5	16	132
muenster	1 ounce	104	9	27	178
Neufchatel	1 ounce	74	6	22	113
Parmesan	1/3 cup	130	9	28	247
pimento	1/4 cup	106	9	27	405
provolone	1 ounce	100	8	20	248
ricotta cheese, regular	1/2 cup	216	16	63	104
part-skim	1/2 cup	170	10	38	153
Roquefort	1 ounce	100	8	45	395
Swiss	1 ounce	110	8	35	75
Cherries, fresh	1/2 cup	45	0	0	1
Chicken, breast, baked					
without skin	3 ounces	190	7	89	86
breast, fried	3 ounces	327	23	89	498
canned	1/2 cup	200	12	91	42
chow mein	1 cup	95	2	15	725
pot pie	1 piece	503	25	13	863
salad	1/2 cup	127	8	28	345
Chili, beef and bean	1 cup	340	15	34	1355
Chow mein noodles	1/2 cup	200	8	0	320
Cocoa powder	1 tbsp.	18	0	0	25
Coconut	4 tbsp.	180	12	0	7
Coffee creamer,					
non-dairy					
liquid	1 tbsp.	20	2	0	12
powder	1 tsp.	11	1	0	4

New And Natural Ways To Your Lower Blood Pressure, Cholesterol, And Stress

Food	Amount	Fat Kcal	Chol (gm)	Sodium (mg)	(mg)
Cole slaw	1 cup	118	8	7	149
Cookies					
animal crackers	5	43	1	4	30
chocolate chip	1	57	8	2	64
Fig Newton	1	50	1	17	35
ginger snaps	3	50	1	0	69
graham cracker	1	55	1	8	95
molasses cookie	1	71	3	7	58
oatmeal cookie	1	80	3	7	69
Oreo cookie	1	49	2	0	63
Peanut butter cookie	1	232	10	0	85
Rice Krispie bar	2 inch x 2 inch	225	10	0	80
shortbread cookie	1	42	2	0	36
sugar cookie	1	98	3	0	109
vanilla wafers	3	51	2	9	28
Cool Whip	1 tbsp.	14	1	0	1
Corn, on-the-cob	1 ear	169	1	0	0
canned	1/2 cup	70	1	0	195
creamed, can	1/2 cup	110	1	0	300
frozen	1/2 cup	70	0	0	0
Crackers (see Snack foods)					
Cranberry, fresh	1 cup	46	0	0	0
juice	3/4 cup	106	0	0	0
Cream, half and half	1 tbsp.	20	2	6	6
heavy	1 tbsp.	52	6	24	6
sour	1 tbsp.	26	3	5	6
whipped	1/2 cup	210	22	80	20
whipping cream, heavy	1 tbsp.	52	6	21	6
light	1 tbsp.	44	5	17	5
Cucumber	1/2 cup	10	0	0	4
Custard	1/2 cup	150	8	139	105
Dates	1/2 cup	220	0	0	1
Donuts, cake	1	160	8	33	210
glazed	1	180	11	16	100
Egg	1	80	6	252	60

New And Natural Ways To Your Lower Blood Pressure, Cholesterol And Stress

Food	Amount	Fat Kcal	Chol (gm)	Sodium (mg)	(mg)
Egg substitute	1/4 cup	25	0	0	80
Egg noodles, cooked	1 cup	220	220	55	15
Figs, fresh	1 piece	80	80	0	2
dried	2	274	274	0	34
Fish					
bass, baked	3 ounces	82	82	68	59
caviar	1 tbsp.	42	42	94	352
cod, baked	3 ounces	180	180	56	115
crab	3 ounces	100	100	100	850
fish sticks	4	200	200	70	115
flounder, baked	3 ounces	200	200	51	235
haddock, baked	3 ounces	180	180	66	195
halibut, baked	3 ounces	175	175	51	86
herring, canned	1/2 cup	208	208	85	74
lobster	3 ounces	90	90	85	205
mackarel, baked	3 ounces	250	250	95	35
mussels	1/4 cup	48	48	16	104
oysters, fresh	6	80	80	60	90
fried	6	138	138	131	116
perch	3 ounces	227	227	55	153
pike	3 ounces	116	116	55	64
red snapper	3 ounces	93	93	55	67
salmon, baked w/butter	3 ounces	189	189	58	116
canned in water	1/2 cup	160	6	75	425
patty, fried	3 ounces	239	12	64	96
smoked	3 ounces	150	8	85	425
sardines	1/4 cup	58	3	28	184
scallops	3 ounces	105	2	53	250
shrimp, boiled	1 cup	100	1	119	250
fried	1 cup	380	19	240	320
sole, baked	3 ounces	141	1	51	235
sushi (raw fish)	3 ounces	93	1	50	67
swordfish, baked	3 ounces	174	6	43	98
trout	3 ounces	196	5	55	61
tuna, canned in oil	3 ounces	176	9	19	535
canned in water	3 ounces	109	2	30	399
low-sodium	3 ounces	106	2	30	33
steak	3 ounces	145	4	60	0
Frankfurter	1	261	17	45	776

New And Natural Ways To Your Lower Blood Pressure, Cholesterol And Stress

Food	Amount	Fat Kcal	Fat (gm)	Chol (mg)	Sodium (mg)
Fruit cocktail, canned, sweetened	1/2 cup	95	0	0	5
Grapefruit, fresh	1/2 medium	40	0	0	1
juice, unsweetened	1 cup	93	0	0	3
Grapes, fresh	1 cup	70	0	0	4
juice	3/4 cup	120	0	0	4
Green chilis, canned	1 tbsp.	14	0	0	0
Green pepper, raw	1/2 cup	15	0	0	10
Greens, collard, cooked	1/3 cup	20	0	0	35
kale, cooked	1 cup	41	0	0	30
spinach, cooked	1/2 cup	20	0	0	50
spinach, raw	1/2 cup	7	0	0	19
Swiss chard, cooked	1/2 cup	15	0	0	60
turnip, cooked	1/2 cup	115	0	0	19
Grits, cooked	1/2 cup	73	0	0	0
Ham, baked, lean	3 ounces	203	8	74	1684
Honey	1 tbsp.	65	0	0	1
Honeydew	1/4 melon	55	0	0	20
Ice cream, regular (10 percent fat)	1/2 cup	135	7	36	60
rich (16 percent fat)	1/2 cup	266	14	72	120
soft serve	1/2 cup	163	10	0	51
Ice milk	1/2 cup	90	3	13	50
Instant breakfast	1 cup	280	8	28	242
Jalapeno pepper, canned	1/4 cup	132	0	0	497
Jam or jelly	1 tbsp.	55	0	0	2
Jello	1/2 cup	70	0	0	0
Kiwi	1 piece	46	0	0	4
Knockwurst	3 ounces	278	23	65	483
Lamb chop, baked	3 ounces	340	28	85	50
roast, baked	3 ounces	160	6	59	60
Lasagna	1 cup	380	12	67	43
Lemon, fresh	1/4 lemon	22	0	0	3
juice	1 tbsp.	5	0	0	0
Lentils	1/3 cup	110	0	0	10
Lettuce	1 cup	6	0	0	6
Lima beans	1/2 cup	95	0	0	2
Lime, fresh	1/4 lime	20	0	0	1

New And Natural Ways To Your Lower Blood Pressure, Cholesterol And Stress

Food	Amount	Fat Kcal	Fat (gm)	Chol (mg)	Sodium (mg)
juice	1 tbsp.	3	0	0	2
Luncheon meats					
bologna	1 ounce	85	8	28	370
pepperoni	1 ounce	139	13	70	492
pimiento loaf	1 ounce	74	6	10	394
salami	1 ounce	130	11	15	350
Macaroni and cheese	1 cup	430	22	42	1085
Macaroni, cooked	1 cup	210	1	0	0
Mandarin oranges, canned	1/2 cup	76	0	0	8
Mango	1 cup	110	0	0	10
Margarine, low-calorie	1 tsp.	16	2	0	49
regular	1	35	4	0	50
unsalted	1 tsp.	35	4	0	0
Marshmallows	1/2 cup	90	0	0	10
Milk, buttermilk, skim	1 cup	90	0	5	318
chocolate, low-fat	1 cup	180	5	5	150
evaporated milk, regular	1 cup	340	20	77	265
evaporated milk, skimmed	1 cup	199	0	10	293
hot chocolate	1 cup	110	3	35	154
low-fat (1 percent fat)	1 cup	102	3	3	122
low-fat (2 percent fat)	1 cup	140	5	5	145
nonfat (dry)	1/4 cup	109	0	6	161
skim	1 cup	90	0	5	125
whole (4 percent fat)	1/2 cup	155	9	34	120
Mixed vegetables, canned	1/2 cup	38	0	0	121
frozen	1/2 cup	54	0	0	45
stir-fried	1/2 cup	59	5	0	17
Mushrooms, canned	1/3 cup	17	0	0	400
fresh	1/2 cup	10	0	0	5
Nectarine, fresh	1	64	0	0	6
Nuts and seeds					
almonds, unsalted	1/4 cup	180	16	0	56
brazil nuts, unslated	1/4 cup	180	19	0	0
cashews, unsalted	1/4 cup	320	26	0	120

New And Natural Ways To Your Lower Blood Pressure, Cholesterol And Stress

Food	Amount	Fat Kcal	(gm)	Chol (mg)	Sodium (mg)
macadamia nuts,					
unsalted	1/4 cup	109	12	0	60
mixed nuts, unsalted	1/4 cup	214	20	0	4
peanuts, salted	1/4 cup	330	28	0	157
peanuts, unsalted	1/4 cup	330	28	0	1
pecans, unsalted	1/4 cup	200	20	0	0
pistachio nuts, salted	1/4 cup	88	8	0	60
sunflower seeds,	1/4 cup	200	17	0	10
unsalted	1/4 cup	200	20	0	0
walnuts, unsalted	1/4 cup	30	0	0	2
Okra, cooked	1/2 cup	35	4	0	150
Olives, black	5	20	3	0	465
green	5	1	0	0	0
Onion, green	1 tbsp.	80	0	0	1
Orange, fresh	1 medium	85	0	0	2
juice	3/4 cup	210	2	63	600
Pancakes (4-inch dia.)	3 medium	60	0	0	4
Papaya	1/2 medium	66	0	0	8
Parsnips	1/2 cup	40	0	0	1
Peach, fresh	1 medium	120	0	0	4
canned, sweetened	2/3 cup	43	0	0	9
canned, unsweetened	2/3 cup	95	8	0	95
Peanut butter, regular	1 tbsp.	95	9	0	5
unsalted	1 tbsp.	100	0	0	3
Pear, fresh	1 medium	65	0	0	2
canned, sweetened	1/2 cup	35	0	0	3
canned, unsweetened	1/2 cup	75	0	0	200
Peas, canned	1/2 cup	55	0	0	90
frozen	1/2 cup	115	0	0	15
split	1/2 cup	15	0	0	1930
Pickles, dill	1 large	50	0	0	200
sweet	1 small	20	0	0	105
relish	1 tbsp.	285	12	40	252
Pie (1 slice),					
banana cream	1/8 pie	264	15	0	273
chocolate cream	1/8 pie	257	14	130	395
lemon meringe	1/8 pie	365	16	0	604

New And Natural Ways To Your Lower Blood Pressure, Cholesterol And Stress

Food	Amount	Fat Kcal	Chol (gm)	Sodium (mg)	(mg)
mincemeat	1/8 pie	334	18	92	177
pecan	1/8 pie				
pumpkin	1/8 pie	320	17	150	325
rhubarb	1/8 pie	190	17	10	432
strawberry	1/8 pie	228	9	10	227
Pimientos, canned	1/4 cup	11	0	0	0
Pineapple, fresh	1 cup	80	0	0	2
canned, sweetened	1 cup	190	0	0	4
canned, unsweetened	1 cup	150	0	0	4
Pizza, cheese (13-inch diameter)	2 slices	340	11	2	900
combination (13-inch diameter)	2 slices	400	17	13	1200
pepperoni (13-inch diameter	2 slices	370	15	27	1000
Plum, fresh	1 large	30	0	0	1
canned, sweetened	1/2 cup	110	0	0	1
canned, unsweetened	1/2 cup	51	0	0	1
Pork chop, broiled	3 1/2 oz.	357	26	77	60
roast, baked	3 ounces	310	24	59	50
Potatoes, au gratin	1/2 cup	95	3	6	529
baked	1 medium	140	0	0	5
French fries	1/2 cup (10 pieces)	220	10	13	120
mashed	1/2 cup	100	5	15	350
tater tots	1/2 cup	200	12	545	545
Prunes, canned	1 cup	245	0	0	6
dried (5 pieces)	1/4 cup	130	0	0	4
Pudding, banana	1/2 cup	241	6	25	11
chocolate	1/2 cup	167	5	65	160
low-calorie	1/2 cup	76	0	0	146
tapioca	1/2 cup	110	4	9	130
vanilla	1/2 cup	140	5	16	85
Quiche (1 slice), cheese	1/8 pie	448	39	305	869
cheese and bacon	1/8 pie	520	42	310	970
Radishes	1/2 cup	7	0	0	10
Raisins	1/4 cup	100	0	0	10

Food	Amount	Fat Kcal	Chol (gm)	Sodium (mg)	(mg)
Raspberries, fresh	1/2 cup	40	0	0	1
frozen	1/2 cup	128	0	0	0
Rhubarb, cooked, sweetened	1/2 cup	190	0	0	2
Rice, brown	2/3 cup	160	1	0	370
white	2/3 cup	150	0	0	2
wild	1 tbsp.	33	0	0	1
Rice-a-Roni	1/3 cup	165	5	13	820
Rice cakes	1 cake	31	0	0	8
Salad dressings					
blue cheese	1 tbsp.	75	8	4	165
blue cheese, low-cal	1 tbsp.	10	1	4	177
French	1 tbsp.	65	6	1	220
French, low-cal	1 tbsp.	22	0	1	128
green goddess	1 tbsp.	68	7	1	150
Italian	1 tbsp.	85	9	1	315
Italian, low-cal	1 tbsp.	15	2	1	118
mayonnaise	1 tbsp.	100	11	8	85
mayonnaise, low-cal	1 tbsp.	50	5	1	100
oil and vinegar	1 tbsp.	71	8	0	0
Ranch or buttermilk	1 tbsp.	53	5	4	185
Russian	1 tbsp.	76	8	0	133
thousand island,	1 tbsp.	80	8	8	110
thousand island, low-cal	1 tbsp.	24	2	2	153
Sauces and condiments					
barbecue	1 tbsp.	15	1	0	130
bearnaise	1 cup	701	68	189	1265
catsup	1 tbsp.	15	0	0	155
chili	1 tbsp.	17	0	0	228
chocolate	2 tbsp.	100	0	2	36
gravy	1/4 cup	164	14	7	720
hollandaise	1/4 cup	361	39	382	400
mustard	1 tsp.	4	0	0	65
picante or salsa	1 1/2 tbsp.	10	0	0	111
soy	2 tbsp.	25	0	0	2665
soy, low-sodium	2 tbsp.	25	0	0	1200
steak	1 tbsp.	18	0	0	149

New And Natural Ways To Your Lower Blood Pressure, Cholesterol And Stress

Food	Amount	Fat Kcal	Chol (gm)	Sodium (mg)	(mg)
tartar	2 tbsp.	75	8	10	100
teriyaki	1 tbsp.	15	0	0	690
white	1/2 cup	200	16	16	475
Worcestershire	1 tsp.	4	0	0	49
Sauerkraut	1/2 cup	20	0	0	880
Sausage, link	1	134	0	0	175
patty	1	112	8	34	418
Polish	3 ounces	276	24	60	744
Scallions	1/4 cup	10	0	0	1
Shallots	1/3 cup	36	0	0	6
Sherbert	1/2 cup	134	1	0	10
Snack foods and crackers					
Cheetos	1 cup	153	10	9	329
corn chips	1 cup	155	10	0	183
peanut butter cracker sandwich	1 sandwich	61	4	3	103
popcorn, air-popped	2 cups	80	1	0	0
popcorn, caramel	2 cups	270	2	0	0
popcorn, cheese	2 cups	130	8	5	280
popcorn, cooked with oil	2 cups	106	5	13	466
potato chips	1 cup	115	8	0	200
pretzels, sticks	50 sticks	109	1	0	875
pretzels, 3-ring	10 rings	120	2	0	500
rice cakes	1 cake	31	0	0	8
Ritz crackers	5 crackers	76	3	8	180
Rykrisp crackers	2 crackers	40	0	0	110
saltines	4 squares	50	2	8	125
saltines,unsalted tops	4 squares	50	2	8	83
shoestring potato sticks	1 cup	152	10	3	280
tortilla chips	1 cup	135	6	0	99
trail mix	1/3 cup	189	10	0	236
Triscuit crackers	2 crackers	60	2	0	90
Wheat thin crackers	4 crackers	70	3	0	120
Soups, bean	1 cup	170	6	10	1010
beef noodle	1 cup	84	3	5	952

New And Natural Ways To Your Lower Blood Pressure, Cholesterol And Stress

Food	Amount	Fat Kcal	Chol (gm)	Sodium (mg)	(mg)
black bean	1 cup	116	2	0	110
broth, beef	1 cup	16	0	0	782
broth, beef low-sodium	1 cup	16	0	0	12
broth, chicken	1 cup	16	0	0	782
broth, chicken low-sodium	1 cup	16	0	0	7
chicken noodle	1 cup	75	2	7	1107
cream of mushroom	1 cup	203	14	20	1076
gazpacho	1 cup	57	2	0	1183
gumbo, chicken	1 cup	200	4	22	970
lentil	1 cup	108	0	0	1038
minestrone	1 cup	83	3	2	911
onion	1 cup	65	2	5	1051
onion, dehydrated	1 cup	21	0	0	636
pea	1 cup	140	3	4	940
potato	1 cup	148	7	22	1060
tomato	1 cup	90	3	4	970
turkey	1 cup	136	4	9	923
vegetable	1 cup	78	4	0	1010
vegetable beef	1 cup	80	2	4	1050
vegetable, chunky	1 cup	122	4	0	1010
won ton	1 cup	92	2	1	2027
Spaghetti, cooked	1 cup	210	1	0	5
Spam	1 ounce	87	7	15	336
Squash (winter), baked	1/2 cup	65	0	0	1
Strawberries, fresh	2/3 cup	35	0	0	1
frozen, sweetened	1/3 cup	160	0	0	2
frozen, unsweetened	2/3 cup	119	0	0	2
Succotash	1 cup	222	2	0	32
Sweet potato or yam, baked	3/4 cup	160	0	0	15
canned	3/4 cup	216	5	10	67
Syrup, corn	1 tbsp.	58	0	0	14
maple	1 tbsp.	50	0	0	2
Taco shell	1 piece	135	6	0	99
Tangerine, fresh	1 medium	46	0	0	2
Tofu	1/2 cup	85	5	0	10
Tofutti	1/2 cup	230	14	0	95

New And Natural Ways To Your Lower Blood Pressure, Cholesterol And Stress

Food	Amount	Fat Kcal	Chol (gm)	Sodium (mg)	(mg)
Tomato, fresh	1/2 cup	25	0	0	4
canned, regular	1/2 cup	25	0	0	155
canned, no salt added	1/2 cup	25	0	0	20
juice	3/4 cup	35	0	0	365
juice, low-sodium	3/4 cup	31	0	0	18
paste	1/2 cup	110	1	0	50
sauce, canned	1/2 cup	43	0	0	656
sauce, canned, no salt added	1/2 cup	43	0	0	25
Tortilla, corn (6-inch diameter)	1	65	1	0	1
flour (8-inch diameter)	1	105	3	0	134
Turkey, dark meat, baked without skin	3 ounces	170	7	64	85
light meat, baked without skin	3 ounces	150	4	64	70
roll, light and dark meat	3 ounces	126	6	48	498
turkey ham	3 ounces	73	3	0	563
Turnips	1/2 cup	20	0	0	25
Veal cutlet	3 ounces	231	13	76	55
patty	3 ounces	298	19	90	51
Waffle	4 in. square	124	5	32	340
Water chestnuts, canned	1/4 cup	20	0	0	5
Watercress	1 cup	5	0	0	20
Watermelon	2 1/4 cup	110	0	0	5
Yogurt, plain nonfat	1 cup	127	68	4	174
frozen	1/2 cup	108	1	0	0
Zucchini, cooked	1 cup	22	0	0	2
raw	1 cup	38	0	0	3

ACUPUNCTURE GLOSSARY

ACUPOINTS--Acupuncture points throughout the body that correspond to specific organs.

ADRENAL GLANDS--Hormone producing (endocrine) glands, located on top of each kidney, responsible for secreting several hormones related to the regulation of blood pressure, including epinephrine and aldosterone.

AEROBIC EXERCISE--Physical activities strenuously performed so as to cause marked temporary increases in respiration and heart rate. These include dynamic exercises and large muscle group activities such as and running.

ALDOSTERONE--A steroid hormone that is released by the adrenal gland and acts on the kidney to promote conservation of sodium and water, thereby raising blood pressure.

ALLOPATHY--Term for standard Western medicine; from the Greek allos (different) and pathein (disease, suffering), thus implying the use of drugs whose effects are different from those of the disease being treated.

ALPHA BLOCKERS--Drugs that lower blood pressure by working with the autonomic nervous system to dilate the blood vessels.

ANAEROBIC EXERCISE--Exercise that draws upon the muscles' own stores of energy and does not require oxygen, such as weight lifting and isometric exercises.

ANGINA PECTORIS--Medical term for chest pain due to coronary heart disease. A condition in which the heart muscle doesn't receive enough blood, resulting in pain in the chest.

ANGIOGRAM--An X-ray picture of blood vessels or chambers of the heart that shows the course of a special fluid called a contrast medium or dye injected into the bloodstream.

ANGIOPLASTY--A procedure sometimes used to inflate (widen) narrowed arteries. A catheter with a deflated balloon on its tip is passed into the narrowed artery segment, the balloon inflated, and the narrowed segment widened.

ANTI-INFLAMMATORY--A substance that soothes inflammation or reduces the inflammatory response of the tissue directly.

AORTA--The large artery that receives blood from the heart's left ventricle and distributes it to the body.

AORTIC VALVE--The heart valve between the left ventricle and the aorta. It has three flaps, or cusps.

ARRHYTHMIA (or DYSRHYTHMIA)--An abnormal rhythm of the heart.

ARTERIOGRAM--An examination of a portion of the circulatory system performed by injecting dye through a catheter into the arteries, thereby forming a map of the blood vessels.

ARTERIOGRAPHY--A testing procedure in which an X-ray opaque dye is injected into the bloodstream, and then pictures are taken and studied to see if the arteries are damaged.

ARTERIOLES--Small, muscular branches of arteries. When they contract, they increase resistance to blood flow, and blood pressure in the arteries increases.

ARTERY--Any one of a series of blood vessels that carry blood from the heart to the various parts of the body. Arteries have thick, elastic walls that can expand as blood flows through them.

ATHEROSCLEROSIS--A form of arteriosclerosis in which the inner layers of artery walls become thick and irregular due to deposits of fat, cholesterol and other substances. This buildup is sometimes called "plaque." As the interior walls of arteries become lined with layers of these deposits, the arteries become narrowed, and the flow of blood through them is reduced.

AUTONOMIC NERVOUS SYSTEM--The part of the nervous system responsible for bodily functions such as the heartbeat, blood pressure, and digestion. It is divided into two divisions, the sympathetic nervous system and the parasympathetic nervous system.

ATRIUM--Either one of the two upper chambers of the heart in which blood collects before being passed to the ventricles.

BACTERIAL ENDOCARDITIS--A bacterial infection of the heart lining or valves. People with abnormal heart valves or congenital heart defects are at increased risk of developing this disease.

BETA BLOCKER--A drug that prevents stimulation of certain receptors of the nerves of the sympathetic nervous system, which would otherwise increase the heart rate.

BIOFEEDBACK--A behavior modification therapy in which people are taught to control bodily functions such as blood pressure through conscious effort.

BLOOD CLOT--A jellylike mass of blood tissue formed by clotting factors in the blood. This clot can then stop the flow of blood from an injury. Blood clots also can form inside an artery whose walls are damaged by atherosclerotic buildup and can cause heart attack or stroke.

BLOOD PRESSURE-The force or pressure exerted by the heart in pumping blood; the pressure of blood in the arteries.

CALCIUM-CHANNEL BLOCKERS--Drugs that keep some calcium from reaching the smooth muscle of the blood vessels, thereby dilating the vessels and lowering arterial pressure.

CALORIE--A unit of measure that represents the amount of energy in foods. The term is also used to represent the amount of energy used by the body for basic body functions and the amount of energy expended through physical activity.

CAPILLARIES--Microscopically small blood vessels between arteries and veins that distribute oxygenated blood to the body's tissues.

CARBOHYDRATE--Organic compounds of carbon, hydrogen, and oxygen, which include starches, cellulose, and sugars, and an important source of energy. All carbohydrates are eventually broken down in the body to glucose, a simple sugar.

CARDIAC--Pertaining to the heart.

CARDIAC ARREST--The stopping of the heartbeat, usually because of interference with the electrical signal (often associated with coronary heart disease).

CARDIOLOGY--The study of the heart and its functions in health and disease.

CARDIOMYOPATHY--A serious disease frequently affecting young people; it involves an inflammation and decreased function in heart muscle. There may be multiple causes including viral infections.

CARDIOPULMONARY RESUSCITATION (CPR)--A combination of chest compression and mouth-to-mouth breathing, this technique is used during cardiac arrest to keep oxygenated blood flowing to the heart muscle and brain until advanced cardiac life support can be started or an adequate heartbeat resumes.

CARDIOVASCULAR--Pertaining to the heart and blood vessels. ("Cardio" means heart; "vascular" means blood vessels.) The circulatory system of the heart and blood vessels is the cardiovascular system.

CARMINATIVE--Term in herbal medicine to denote plants that help the digestive system to work properly by soothing any inflammation that might be present and removing any excess gas in the digestive tract.

CAROTID ARTERY--A major artery in the neck.

CATHETERIZATION--Process of examining the heart byintroducing a thin tube (catheter) into a vein or artery and passing it into the heart.

CENTRAL NERVOUS SYSTEM--The brain and the spinal cord, which are responsible for the integration of all neurological functions.

CHANNELS--Also called meridians; in traditional Chinese medicine, the invisible pathways of qi both on the surface of and within the body.

CHINESE MEDICINE--A philosophy and methodology of health and medicine developed in ancient China.

CHOLESTEROL--A fat-like substance found in animal tissue and present only in foods from animal sources such as whole milk dairy products, meat, fish, poultry, animal fats and egg yolks.

CIRCULATORY SYSTEM--Pertaining to the heart, blood vessels and the circulation of the blood.

CONGENITAL--Refers to conditions existing at birth.

CONGENITAL HEART DEFECTS--Malformation of the heart or of its major blood vessels present at birth.

CONGESTIVE HEART FAILURE--The inability of the heart to pump out all the blood that returns to it. This results in blood backing up in the veins that lead to the heart and sometimes in fluid accumulating in various parts the body.

CORONARY ARTERIES--Two arteries arising from the aorta that arch down over the top of the heart, branch, and provide blood to the heart muscle.

CORONARY ARTERY DISEASE--Conditions that cause narrowing of the coronary arteries so blood flow to the heart muscle is reduced.

CORONARY BYPASS SURGERY--Surgery to improve blood supply to the heart muscle. This surgery is most often performed when narrowed coronary arteries reduce the flow of oxygen-containing blood to the heart itself.

CORONARY CARE UNIT--A specialized facility in a hospital or emergency mobile unit that's equipped with monitoring devices and staffed with trained personnel. It's designed specifically to treat coronary patients.

CORONARY HEART DISEASE--Disease of the heart caused by atherosclerotic narrowing of the coronary arteries likely to produce angina pectoris or heart attack.

CORONARY THROMBOSIS--Formation of a clot in one of the arteries that conduct blood to the heart muscle. Also called coronary occlusion.

DEFIBRILLATOR--An electronic device that helps reestablish normal contraction rhythms in a malfunctioning heart.

DETOXIFICATION--In Ayurveda, the process of removing toxins from the body.

DIABETES--A disease in which the body doesn't produce or properly use insulin. Insulin is needed to convert sugar and starch into the energy needed in daffy life. The full name for this condition is diabetes mellitus.

DIASTOLE--The interval between heartbeats when the heart relaxes and fills with blood. The diastolic reading in a blood pressure measurement is the lower number.

DIURETIC--A drug that increases the rate at which urine forms by promoting the excretion of water and salts.

DOSHAS--In Ayurvedic medicine, the three basic biological types which determine an individual's constitution.

ECHOCARDIOGRAPHY--A diagnostic method in which pulses of sound are transmitted into the body and the echoes returning from the surfaces of the heart and other structures are electronically plotted and recorded to produce a "picture" of the heart's size, shape and movements.

ELECTROCARDIOGRAM (ECG or EKG)--A graphic record of electrical impulses produced by the heart.

ENDOCRINE SYSTEM--A network of glands that secrete hormones into the bloodstream. Hormones help to control body processes including digestion, circulation, reproduction, and growth.

ENDORPHINS--Natural substances produced by the body which function as natural painkillers.

ENZYME--A complex chemical capable of speeding up specific biochemical processes in the body.

EPINEPHRINE--Also called adrenaline. A hormone secreted by the adrenal glands that increases the heart rate and constricts blood vessels.

ESSENTIAL FATTY ACIDS--Unsaturated fatty acids which cannot be synthesized in the body and are considered essential for maintaining health.

ESSENTIAL OIL--Concentrated, pure aromatic essence extracted from plants.

EXCESS CONDITION--In traditional Chinese medicine, a condition in which qi, blood, or body fluids are disordered and accumulate in channels or elsewhere in the body.

FAT--An essential nutrient, the principal form in which energy is stored in the body.

FIGHT-OR-FLIGHT RESPONSE--The body's response to perceived danger or stress, involving the release of hormones and subsequent rise in heart rate, blood pressure, and muscle tension.

FIVE PHASES THEORY--In Chinese medicine, a way of looking at the body and the universe that explains the interaction between them.

FREE RADICALS--Molecules that are highly reactive and potentially destructive to the body.

GLUCOSE--The most common simple sugar; essential source of energy for the body.

HEART ATTACK--Death of, or damage to part of theheart muscle due to an insufficient blood supply.

HEART-LUNG MACHINE--An apparatus that oxygenates and pumps blood to the body while a person's heart is opened for surgery.

HEART RATE--The number of times the heart beats (contracts and releases) each minute.

HEMOGLOBIN--The oxygen-carrying red pigment component of the red blood cells. Hemoglobin transports oxygen to the body tissue and removes carbon dioxide.

HEREDITY--The genetic transmission of a particular quality or trait from parent to offspring.

HIGH BLOOD PRESSURE--A chronic increase in blood pressure above normal range.

HIGH DENSITY LIPOPROTEIN (HDL)--A carrier of cholesterol believed to transport cholesterol away from the tissues and to the liver, where it can be removed from the bloodstream.

HOLISTIC--Pertaining to the whole body; treatment of disease by taking into consideration every part of the body, not only the presenting symptoms, to bring the internal environment into balance.

HOMEOPATHIC REMEDY--A remedy, selected on the basis of the similarity of its symptoms, that produces a reaction in a patient that stimulates an immune system response.

HORMONE--Internal secretion that is transported by the bloodstream to various organs to regulate or modify vital bodily functions and processes.

HYPERLIPIDEMIA--Excessive fats in the blood.

HYPERTENSION--Same as High Blood Pressure.

INFARCTION--The death of tissue that occurs when the blood supply to a localized part of the body is blocked.

INSULIN--A hormone produced and secreted by the pancreas; necessary for proper metabolism, particularly of carbohydrates and the uptake of glucose.

ISCHEMIA--Decreased blood flow to an organ, usually due to constriction or obstruction of an artery.

KIDNEYS--The two bean-shaped glands, situated at the back of the abdomen, that regulate salt volume and composition of thebody fluids by filtering the blood and eliminating waste throughthe production of urine.

LAW OF SIMILARS--The principle that "like shall be cured by like" that forms the basis of homeopathy; the proper remedy for a patient's disease is that substance that is capable of producing, in a healthy person, symptoms similar to those from which the patient suffers.

LIMBIC SYSTEM--A group of brain structures that influence the endocrine and autonomic nervous systems.

LIPIDS--Fats, steroids, phospholipids, and glycolipids; fat or fatlike substances.

LIPOPROTEIN--The combination of lipid surrounded by a protein; the protein makes it soluble in blood.

LOW DENSITY LIPOPROTEIN (LDL)--The main carrier of "harmful" cholesterol in the blood.

MANIPULATION--Technique used in chiropractic therapy to adjust the spine, joints, and other tissue.

MERIDIANS--In traditional Chinese medicine, the fourteen channels in the body through which qi runs.

METHIONINE--An essential amino acid.

MOBILIZATION--A technique of chiropractic therapy that gently increases the range of movement of a joint.

MONOUNSATURATED FAT--A type of fat found in many foods but predominantly in canola, olive, and peanut oil and avocados.MOXA--Dried mugwort leaves used in traditional Chinese medicine; placed on the end of needles, then lighted and held near an acupuncture point to warm and tonify qi.

MUSCULOSKELETAL SYSTEM--Pertaining to the muscles and skeleton.

MYOCARDIAL ISCHEMIA--Deficient blood flow to part of the heart muscle.

MYOCARDIUM--The muscular wall of the heart. It contracts to pump blood out of the heart and then relaxes as the heart refills with returning blood.

NEUROTRANSMITTERS--Substances that transmit messages to, from, and within the brain and other body tissues.

NICOTINE--A chemical substance derived from

tobacco that affects blood pressure and pulse rate.

NOREPINEPHRINE--A hormone secreted by the adrenal gland that raises blood pressure by constricting small blood vessels and increasing blood flow through the coronary arteries.

OBESITY--The condition of being significantly overweight. Usually applied to a condition of 20 percent or more over ideal body weight. Obesity puts a strain on the heart and can increase the chance of developing high blood pressure and diabetes.

OPEN HEART SURGERY--Surgery performed on the opened heart while the bloodstream is diverted through a heart-lung machine.

OXYGENATION--To supply or combine with oxygen.

PACEMAKER--An electrical device that can substitute for a defective natural pacemaker or conduction pathway. The artificial pacemaker controls the heart's beating by emitting a series of rhythmic electrical discharges.

PALPATION--Physical examination of the body using hands to feel for abnormalities.

PANCREAS--The gland situated behind the stomach that secretes a number of substances important for digestion, including the hormone insulin.

PARASYMPATHETIC NERVOUS SYSTEM--The division of the nervous system that, when stimulated, slows heart rate, lowers blood pressure, and slows breathing.

PITTA--An Ayurvedic dosha.

PLAQUE--A deposit of fatty (and other) substances in the inner of the artery wall characteristic of atherosclerosis.

PLATELET--Component of the blood involved in blood clotting.

POLYUNSATURATED FATS--Oils of vegetable origin such as corn, safflower, sunflower, and soybean oil that are liquid at room temperature.

POTENCY--The dilution of homeopathic remedies to increase their effectiveness, thus giving them their therapeutic value.

PREMATURE VENTRICULAR CONTRACTION (PVC)--Irregular heartbeat that starts in the ventricles.

PULMONARY--Pertaining to the lungs.

QI--In traditional Chinese medicine, the life-force or energy of the body and the universe that circulates through the body's channels.

QI STAGNATION--Any blockage of energy in the body that interrupts the body's natural functions or the healing process.

RHEUMATIC HEART DISEASE--Damage done to the heart, particularly the heart valves, by one or more attacks of rheumatic fever.

RISK FACTOR--When referring to the heart and blood vessels, a risk factor is associated with an increased chance of developing cardiovascular disease, including stroke.

SATURATED FATS--Types of fat found in foods of animal origin and a few of vegetable origin; they are typically solid at room temperature.

SCLEROSIS--An abnormal thickening or hardening of the arteries and other vessels.

SEDENTARY--Engages in minimal or no physical activity.

SHEN--In traditional Chinese medicine, the "spirit" or consciousness, which both originates and forms the outward expression of human life.

SILENT ISCHEMIA--Episodes of ischemia that aren't accompanied by pain.

SODIUM--A mineral essential to life found in nearly all plant and animal tissue. Table salt (sodium chloride) is nearly half sodium.

STRESS--Bodily or mental tension within a person resulting from his or her response to physical, chemical, or emotional factors. Stress can refer to physical exertion as well as mental anxiety.

STROKE (also called Apoplexy, Cerebrovascular Accident, or Cerebral Vascular Accident)--Loss of muscle function, vision, sensation or speech resulting from brain cell damage caused by an insufficient supply of blood to part of the brain.

SUBLUXATION--In chiropractic, a term used to explain a misalignment of spinal vertebrae.

SUCCUSSION--The forceful shaking of liquid homeopathic remedies that allows the permeation of the medicinal substance into the alcohol tincture.

SUDDEN CARDIAC DEATH--Death that occurs unexpectedly and instantaneously or shortly after the onset of symptoms. The most common underlying reason for patients dying suddenly is cardiovascular disease, in particular coronary heart disease.

SYMPATHETIC NERVOUS SYSTEM--The division of the autonomic nervous system responsible for such actions as blood pressure, salivation, and digestion; works in balance with the parasympathetic nervous system.

SYMPTOMS--Observable or internal changes in the mental, emotional, and physical condition of a person; in holistic medicine, symptoms are the external proof of an internal imbalance.

SYSTOLE--The contraction of the heart muscle; systolicpressure is the greater of the two numbers in a blood pressure reading.

SYSTOLIC BLOOD PRESSURE--The highest blood pressure measured in the arteries. It occurs when the heart contracts with each heartbeat.

TAO--The course of nature and ways of nature; a Chinese term denoting the universe as an undifferentiated whole.

THALLIUM SCAN--A medical diagnostic test in which thallium, a radioactive isotope, is injected in a vein during exercise and then scanned with a special instrument in an effort to detect myocardial ischemia.

THROMBOSIS--The formation or presence of a blood clot (thrombus) inside a blood vessel or cavity of the heart.

TINCTURE--An alcoholic solution of a medicinal substance.

TONIFY--In Chinese medicine, to nourish, augment, and invigorate; to add to the supply of qi and to promote the proper functioning and balance in the body.

TOXIN--Substance that is harmful or poisonous to the body.

TRANSIENT ISCHEMIA ATTACK (TIA)--A temporary stroke-likeevent that lasts for only a short time and is caused by atemporarily blocked blood vessel.

TRIGLYCERIDE--A fat that comes from food or is made in the body from other energy sources such as carbohydrates.

ULTRASOUND--High-frequency sound vibrations, not audible to the human ear, used in medical diagnosis.

VASCULAR--Pertaining to blood vessels.

VASOCONSTRICTOR--An agent that causes blood vessels to narrow, thereby causing a decrease in blood flow.

VASODILATOR--An agent that causes the blood vessels to widen, thereby increasing blood flow. VEIN--Any one of a series of blood vessels of the vascular system that carries blood from various parts of the body back to the heart.

VENTRICLE--One of the two lower chambers of the heart.

VITAL FORCE--In homeopathy, the intangible energy that animates all living creatures and mediates their physical, emotional, and intellectual responses to external stress.

YANG ORGANS--In Chinese medicine, the yang organs include the intestines, gallbladder, and skin.

YIN ORGANS--In Chinese medicine, the yin organs are dense, internal organs such as the heart, liver, lungs, kidneys, and bones.

YIN-YANG--Chinese concept that describes all existence in terms of states or conditions that are different but mutually dependent; traditional Chinese medicine aims to restore balance to these contrasting aspects of the body and mind.